The Dawn Phenomenon ™

Diabetes or Super Wellness?

Life Changing Health Coaching:
An Introduction

G. E. Frazier, CHC

©2014 by G. E. Frazier, CHC
All rights reserved. Published 2015.
CreateSpace

ISBN-13: 978-1505330892
ISBN-10: 1505330890

Library of Congress Control Number: 2014921550
CreateSpace Independent Publishing Platform
North Charleston, South Carolina

I dedicate this book to you, the reader. You are busy. I know, and I really want you to read this book because it will change your life. So I trimmed it down so you can get through it in one sitting. Then call me or e-mail me, and I will look after you. Guaranteed.

DawnPhenomenon@GEFrazier.com
http://www.GEFrazier.Com
http://www.Facebook.com/GeraldFrazierHC

I also dedicate my book to my love, Melanie Savin. You show the patience of Job always, but especially in these last three years.

CONTENTS

PART I: NOVEMBER 17, 2011 — 1

1—THE WAKE-UP CALL
November 17, 2011, at 11:17 a.m. — 3

2—INTRODUCTION AND ACTIONS
IN THREE WORDS — 9

3—THE DISCOVERY OF THE CENTURY
November 17, 2011, at noon — 13

4—TWITTER PROFILE
November 18, 2011, at 11:00 p.m. — 17
Exercise found on the internet — 18
Water — 20
"Sleep is the best meditation" –Dalai Lama XIV — 22

5—HONOR YOUR ANCESTORS
November 20, 2011, at 9:30 a.m. — 25
The fasting blood glucose test — 30
But i have proof — 32

6—STANDARD AMERICAN DIET (SAD)
November 21, 2011, at 9:00 a.m. — 37

PART II: DECEMBER 2011   *49*

7—PRIMARY FOODS
December 1, 2011, at 4:45 a.m.   *51*
December 2, 2011   *54*
December 3, 2011   *54*
December 4, 2011   *54*
December 6, 2011   *54*
December 9, 2011   *55*

8—"WHAT IS TRUTH?" –PONTIUS PILATE IN JOHN 18:38
December 17, 2011, at 9:00 a.m.   *57*

9—HORMONE D
December 17, 2011, at 5:30 p.m.   *65*

10—EARTHING
December 18, 2011   *69*

11—COCONUT OIL
December 19, 2011   *73*

12—A PARTIAL LIST OF L-GAAT, LIES - GENERALLY ACCEPTED AS TRUE
December 20, 2011   *77*

13—NURSE MARTI AND THE ADA
December 21, 2011   *81*

14—SIR LANCE-A-LOT, FINGER-POKIN', AND I TEST UNDER "100"
December 27, 2011   *85*

CONTENTS

15—CINNAMON   *89*
December 31, 2011, at midnight

PART III: 2012 AND 2013   *93*

16—JOURNALS, TABLES, AND CHARTS, OH MY   *95*
January 19, 2012, at midnight

17—MY FINAL DOCTOR'S VISIT
January 20, 2012, at 5:20 a.m.   *109*
Regarding flu shots: *110*

18—FURTHER STUDY AND I FIND A NEW CAREER
July 1, 2012   *115*

PART IV: 2014 AND WAY BEYOND   *119*

19—GRADUATION
July 1, 2014   *121*

EPILOGUE   *127*

REFERENCES AND CONCLUDING THOUGHTS   *129*

ABOUT THE AUTHOR   *133*

PREFACE

Richard Bach an American writer, widely known as the author of the hugely popular 1970s best-sellers Jonathan Livingston Seagull and Illusions: The Adventures of a Reluctant Messiah, among others. said, "A professional writer is an amateur who didn't quit." Look at me: I didn't quit. According to Mr. Bach, that makes me a professional writer. One percent, of the population, write and publish a book. I recommend that you write your story and become part of the 1 percent. I am looking forward to reading your story.

"Speak to the reader. Look into his soul and write." –G. E. Frazier

I sincerely hope that you enjoy reading this book as much as I enjoyed writing it.

ACKNOWLEDGMENTS

I thank Brian Tracy, Joshua Rosenthal, Lindsey Smith, and Carmen Kanazawa, CHC, for their encouragement. It was Carmen who kept me writing when she told me, "I think you have a talent in writing." We shall see. I thank my associates, Douglas Barker, EA, and Steve Arsulich, EA, of O'Connor's Tax Service. Their support allowed me the time necessary to complete this book. I thank my son, Jerry, for his help with the cover and his general encouragement. I thank my youngest son, Omar, for his encouragement and for his help with the website and the book launch. My family always raises my spirits and reminds me that laughter is the best medicine. Good cheer and humor is a big part of health and wellness.

Therefore, I begin this book by stating that it is an Unauthorized Autobiography. In order to tell an interesting story certain literary license is taken, and composites are drawn. It is still based on true events. However, this story is filtered through my memory and memories are always shaded by the one doing the remembering. It is in this sense a fictional book with fictitious characters. Any resemblance these characters may have to actual persons living or sleeping is purely coincidental.

Finally, I appreciate you and all the readers of this book. I thank each and every one of you: Thank you. Thank you. Thank you. Thank you. Thank you. No, thank you. Thank you. I mean it, thank you. Thank you. Thank you. Thank you. Thank you. Thank you. Thank you. Thanks a million. Showing gratitude and expressing appreciation is very good for my health. Thank you. Thank you. Thank you. Thank you. Thank you. Think THANKS, thank you. Thank you.

And thank you. ... Thankyouthankyouthankyou. ThankYou. ... Thankyouverymuch!

Diabetes is a serious subject; a little humor is going to make it bearable: you know, a spoonful of sugar makes the medicine go down. Only, from now on we will be substituting honey for sugar. A spoonful of honey makes the medicine go down. Only my solution is drugless, so there is no medicine in the typical sense of the word. Therefore, it goes like this: a spoonful of honey without medicine to go down. - Sweet.

A Norwegian study* tracked 2,015 cancer patients over several years. Those with a healthy sense of humor were 70 percent less likely to die than those with a weak sense of humor.
*Sala Horowitz, *Alternative and Complementary Therapies.* August 2009 15(4): 196-202.

PART I
NOVEMBER 17, 2011

1
The Wake-Up Call

November 17, 2011, at 11:17 a.m.

"You.

Are.

Diabetic.

And your diabetes is out of control."

Imagine hearing this from your doctor, unexpectedly, as I just did. Next, without the slightest hint of a pause, and without looking down, Dr. Smith, my doctor, pulls out his Rx pad and flips it open. He does this all in one rapid, yet fluid motion—a matter-of-fact next step. Something he has done thousands of times before. The sound it makes seems louder than it really is by the unexpected nature of it, so that it shatters the silence in his exam room like a foghorn on a clear night. However, it isn't the sound of the Rx pad that startles me; it is the myriad of implications, some real, some imagined.

My doctor had been looking me straight in the eye; now his gaze drops to the newly arrived Rx pad, which he is holding in his left hand, while his right hand instinctively retrieves his black fountain pen from the breast pocket of his white smock. I sit in front of him helpless, frozen in fear. His black pen is now deftly whizzing across the face of the first of many prescriptions. Exotic names of medicines race through his well-trained medical mind like so many hot fluffy white kernels of freshly popped corn releasing themselves from a popcorn popper.

I know I have a shocked look on my face. This is not at all what I had expected. I came in for a routine checkup. I am not sick! And certainly, I do not have an incurable degenerative disease. What did the doctor just say, "Out of control?" That implies it can be controlled, but not cured: a problem to be managed by taking Rx drugs for the rest of my life.

Stunned or not, I finally hear myself vehemently protesting, "I will control it with diet and exercise…and cinnamon."

I still don't know where the idea of cinnamon came from. Heck, I don't know where the idea of diet and exercise came from. The only thing I know about being a diabetic is that he, or she, has to take more and more drugs, while still getting worse and worse over the length of his, or her, shortened life. Word on the street is that diabetes shortens a person's life by twenty years.

Dr. Smith is obviously skeptical as he finally allows himself to say, "You take your…cinnamon…and I'll see you back here in… six weeks."

"OK." I quickly respond as Dr. Smith continues.

"In the meantime the nurse can give you your flu shot."

"No flu shot, Thank you."

On the way to the reception window the nurse offers me a flu shot anyway.

"No, thank you."

The receptionist is pleasant as she matter-of-factly states, "For today's office visit, there is a ten-dollar co-pay."

I pay and head for the door when I hear her call out to me, "Oh wait, you haven't had your flu shot yet."

"No thanks."

~·~

This day, November 17, 2011, is a day I will never forget. In a daze, I leave my doctor's office. My car attracts me to it without having to think about where I had parked it. I am too busy reflecting back on my lifelong habit of drinking Coca-Cola and other soft drinks.

When thirsty, I always look for "The Real Thing." MacDonald's has an ongoing special: "64 ounces for 49 cents." So most days, I buy two "64 ounce Cokes." The taste is so good with my cheeseburger lunch. Two times sixty-four ounces is—wow—a gallon. Imagine drinking a gallon of sugar every day. I decide right then and there: "*I have stopped my soda-sugar addiction.*"

Questions are swirling around in my head, preventing my mind from clearing; however, one thing is clear: I have to begin a serious inquiry into nutrition. Since I know nothing about nutrition, it is, for me, a journey into the unknown—a voyage of discovery that my very life depends upon. Where this journey will lead, and when it will end, I do not know.

There is not a shadow of a doubt in my mind that I have just now given up sugar for good. However, will that alone be enough to get me back to good health? I am determined to find out.

~·~

Feeling compelled to ask, I google: "What is diabetes?" The Internet says, "There are at least five types: type I, one and one half, II, two and one half, and type III, and something called the Dawn Phenomenon."

I am vaguely aware of types I and II, but the others I have never even heard of. After hours of research, I find that the label diabetes is not very specific. It is a hormone called insulin that we should research.

Type I diabetes is an insulin deficiency from childhood, type one and one half is adult onset insulin defiency, and type II is an insulin resistance. Type two and one half is a temporary insulin deficiency or resistance during pregnancy. Type III is too much glucose in the brain resulting in Alzheimer's, according to some cutting edge researchers. And then there is the Dawn Phenomenon.

~·~

You yourself may be a Dawn Phenomenon. There are about 70,000,000 of us in the United States alone, and we are in danger of being misdiagnosed as diabetic, and then given prescription drugs to treat the symptoms of diabetes.

However, these drugs have equally serious side effects, and the worst part is they do not cure diabetes and may make it worse in the long run. The medical establishment is interested in selling drugs to treat the symptoms; it is not interested in curing the disease. In 2012 alone, the revenue from diabetes drugs was $245 billion. Let me break that down for you. It looks more formidable in numbers, $245,000,000,000. It also looks like a formidable and terrible conflict of interest for Big Pharma.

These drugs Big Pharma profits from, control the symptoms of diabetes so you can continue on with your same lifestyle—the same lifestyle that got you into poor health in the first place. After that, it was your poor health that caused your diabetes. It is poor health that causes most diseases including diabetes, as you and I are about to learn.

What if you changed your lifestyle, instead of taking their costly drugs? Just say no to drugs. - Just saying.

~·~

As we gain experience, our knowledge and understanding is broadened. As reasoning empathetic humans, we gain experience in two ways, either directly or vicariously by hearing or reading someone else's experience. I am confident that you will benefit from hearing about my experience. And that is enough to compel me to bring you the following problem and solution— so that truth may prevail and set us free.

The problem: Worldwide there are hundreds of millions of us walking time bombs, not knowing that we have a lifestyle that is aging us faster than normal. You could experience the same wake-up call that I just did. If you do, my hope is that you will remember this book and not anguish as much as I did, because you will know what to do to keep it from becoming a life sentence.

I feel this information will help you and many of those hundreds of millions. Since I have this valuable information inside my head and heart, I have a moral obligation to pass it on to you.

In order to fulfill my moral obligation, I offer you this book in the hope that you will find the solution that became so clear to me. I wrote this book to give you this solution. I found out, after many hours self monitoring, journal keeping, and researching, that I need not worry. What I need to do is to live my life in harmony with the fact that I am a Dawn Phenomenon.

And yet this book is so much more than that...

It is a multidimensional book for actions...

2
Introduction and Actions

IN THREE WORDS

You can encapsulate this book *in three words*: Honor your ancestors. Just as imitation is the highest form of flattery, the highest expression of honor is to learn from your ancestors and copy them. I can explain that in nine paragraphs. Then these nine paragraphs are explained by the rest of this book:

Dawn Phenomenon is an actual medical term. It refers to a survival mechanism that has evolved down to you. It gives you energy in the morning, energy enough to catch your breakfast. Having above-average glucose, sugar, in our blood for energy in the morning does not make us diabetic.

ACTION: First thing in the morning, expend energy with twenty minutes of intermittent exercise, then within thirty minutes eat a high protein breakfast.

Dawn Phenomenon is a miracle of rejuvenation. Each night your body rests and repairs itself, a testament to your body's ability to take care of itself, to heal itself, to renew itself, and to prepare you for the next day.

ACTION: Get eight hours sleep.

Dawn Phenomenon is an awakening of the human healing spirit innate in you.
ACTION: Trust your body.

Dawn Phenomenon is a dawning of the phenomenal human body. Your body has the self wisdom and innate ability of self-preservation and self-healing…*if* given the food your body needs at the proper times and in the correct amounts. The right food is a variety of natural, local, seasonal, organic, whole foods.
ACTION: Find good food.

Dawn Phenomenon is a dawning in the minds of people that they have been too trusting and were subsequently lied to and taken advantage of by people with ulterior motives.
ACTION: Question everything, especially authority.

Dawn Phenomenon is a dawning in the morals of people to the idea of self-responsibility for their own health…and for controlling their own lives. You, and only you, hold your very own key to your own health and happiness. Freedom with responsibility is liberty.
ACTION: Guard your liberty.

Dawn Phenomenon holds the promise of expanding knowledge and of holding others responsible and accountable for recognizing and telling the truth, the whole truth, and nothing but the truth. Demand reasonable proof when someone tries to sell you a bill of goods. "Just the facts ma'am."
ACTION: Demand reasonable proof; check it out on the Internet.

Introduction and Actions

Dawn Phenomenon holds out hope for a better tomorrow.
ACTION: Have faith. True hope is well-placed faith.

Dawn Phenomenon is a wellness movement born of a ripple effect.
ACTION: Join us. Let's make it a tidal wave.

My hope is that this *phenomenon* will *dawn* on you, and you will join us in making the ideas in this book a tidal wave, a tidal wave of truth. I do not have the whole truth; like you, I am a seeker of truth. Here is hoping that we will soon become an army of truth seekers.

Let's begin with a major paradigm shift, a fundamental scientific discovery in 1993…

3
The Discovery of the Century

November 17, 2011, at noon

For the first touchstone on our voyage, we have to go back to three medical studies conducted in 1993. They were published later in a prestigious medical journal. The citations are in the References section at the end of this book.

The results should have turned the medical establishment upside down. These studies proved that the scientific basis, for our current medical practices, is flawed.

Currently, medical doctors treat the symptoms of a disease rather than treating the patient.

Currently, medical doctors diagnose the disease then: Cut it out, drug it, or poison it, based on the theory that

Disease causes poor health.

In 1993 that theory was proven *false*, and a new theory was proven *true*:

Poor health causes disease.

In other words, poor health causes disease.

Say it with me: "Poor health causes disease." Not the other way round.

Disease may make your poor health worse, but disease did not create your original poor health. Your original poor health came first, before the disease. It is likely that poor health builds up over a number of years of neglect. Finally, your body gives in to a pathogen or it turns on itself...something to get your attention. What better way to get your attention than by causing you to experience dis-ease? And that is the way to think of disease. You and your body are no longer at ease; you're at dis-ease.

Think about the cause and effect relationship: If your goal is good health, then "curing" the symptoms of your disease does nothing to improve the underlying poor health that caused your disease in the first place. "Curing" the symptoms is like silencing a fire alarm without putting out the fire.

Therefore, before you contract a disease like diabetes, consciously improve your health. Put yourself in good health. This removes the cause of disease. Without a cause, there can be no disease.

Attempts to eliminate the effect (a disease) without addressing the cause (poor health) have failed miserably. Now a scientific theory exists to explain *why*:

1. Why there is no silver bullet, gene splice, or super chemotherapy to make us healthy by eliminating disease;
2. Why diseases are increasing, despite our heroic fund raising efforts, such as walks, runs, rides, telethons, etc.; and
3. Why throwing money at the diseases hasn't worked and never will work.

Out of necessity, I am learning what does work. Out of the need to cure myself of diabetes, which I will do no matter how long it takes.

In the pages ahead I will chronicle my journey to health. Come along and learn from my successes and from my missteps.

My fervent desire is that you will avoid being one of those diagnosed with diabetes. If current health trends persist, your chances are one in three. One third of all US adults will have diabetes by the year 2015, according to the CDC. http://www.diabetes.org/diabetes-basics/statistics/cdc-infographic.html As of 2014 we are on track to hit that target. These citations are also in the References section at the end of this book.

On our journey ahead we will learn how to protect ourselves from diabetes—in fact from most deadly diseases—and do so without dangerous and costly prescription drugs.

Keep in mind this paradigm shift. It should change our current thinking about health, wellness, and all disease, not just diabetes. Recall that it was Albert Einstein who warned us that we cannot solve today's problems with the same thinking that created them. This recent emphasis on health and wellness is revolutionary. It brings new hope for healthy longevity.

And more than that, it has always been a dream of mine to live, and to remain healthy, until the age of 120.

If you look at my Twitter profile you will see the following proclamation ...

4
Twitter Profile

November 18, 2011, at 11:00 p.m.

"U.S. Constitutionalist, Lover of Yahweh & life He gave me. I Plan 2 live 2 age 120, then B shot by jealous husband while tryng 2 escape thru bedrm window"

Pardon the abbreviations. Twitter only gives you 154 spaces for a profile, so I had to abbreviate.

You get a mere 140 spaces for a tweet. The abbreviations used by tweeters fill a whole book. Really...I have seen the book. ROFLOL, RollOnFloorLaughOutLoud.

Hoping to find comfort and solace, I reach out to my Twitter followers.

12:31 am 19 Nov., 2011, I tweet the following abbreviated tweet:

"My dream of living a healthy life to age 120 is in jeoprty. Ive been diagnosed diabetic. Ive been researching, its a complcated condition."

1:13 am I get a reply:

"19 Nov., 2011 you can lead perfectly normal life with diabetes, but you must keep on top of it."

Gee thanks. You sound like my doctor telling me, "You must manage it." How about curing diabetes? How do I cure it?

Well… On Thursday, December 1st, I am booked on Hawaiian Airlines to fly to Hawaii. I think to myself, *I had better get my act together by then.*

~·~

The phone rings.

"Hello."

Maria, the receptionist from my doctor's office, says, "I see here on your chart that you haven't had your flu shot yet. When can you come in for that?"

"No, thank you."

"Well, you have an appointment with Marti Sharon, RN. She will explain everything you need to know about diabetes. Be there ten minutes early please."

"When is my appointment?"

"Your appointment is 2:00 p.m. Thursday, December 1st."

As I hang up the phone, I think to myself, *"The universe is playing with me. I'll bet I don't even have diabetes at all."*

I call Marti Sharon's office and change my appointment to December 21. Hopefully, she will give me some answers then. But I can't wait that long; I have to search the Internet now.

EXERCISE FOUND ON THE INTERNET

One of the first doctors I come across on the Internet is Dr. Mercola. He has a lot of information about fitness and about diabetes. I learn from him that exercise is crucial to balancing your blood glucose (sugar). If you have excess glucose in your

Twitter Profile

blood the best way to reduce it is to burn it up by exercising, but not just any exercising. The latest studies advise against long bouts of aerobic exercise. Seems it's not good for your heart.

Dr. Mercola on his website explains that each muscle set is a set of three different types of muscle fibers. Some are slow muscle fibers. Some are medium speed. Some of your muscle fibers are fast working. We need to exercise each of these for an effective bodybuilding workout. However, to quickly gain the health benefits of exercise then exercising the "fast" muscle fibers is the fastest way to do your workout. Twenty to thirty minutes every other day is all it takes. I start with five minutes on the elliptical machine. This device monitors your heart rate, making it easy to know how you are doing as you warm up.

You can find Dr. Mercola on the Internet at Fitness.Mercola.com where he shows you how he uses these machines. Or you can hire a personal trainer for about $99 for three or four forty-five minute sessions.

My gym has a circuit, twenty weight machines arranged in a circle. It only takes me ten to fifteen minutes to complete the circuit with thirty to forty-five seconds on each machine. Once you get the hang of it, it is fun.

That's it for your aerobics and your weight training. The best time to do this is the first thing every other morning. Don't fret if you miss a morning. It is never too late. I've gone to the gym at 10:00 p.m., and it is less crowded then.

Next is your two-mile walk every other day.

Make it fun and mix it up a bit. Go to the gym one day, and then go for a walk the next day. Alternating that way keeps exercising from becoming monotonous; I am all about variety.

With all this exercise I am feeling better already, but a little thirsty. So I am told on the Internet that I should drink water.

WATER

Doesn't everyone need eight glasses of water daily? No! That is an urban myth. In <u>a 2011 article published in the *British Medical Journal*</u>, "Margaret McCartney debunked the eight glasses a day myth and noted that one water advocacy group in Europe, Hydration for Health, is not only sponsored by, but was actually created by food giant Danone. Under the company's expansive culinary umbrella? Volvic, Evian, and Badoit bottled waters." http://theweek.com/article/index/248725/where-did-the-8-glasses-of-water-a-day-myth-come-from Accessed 12/27/14.

The myth didn't originate with the Bible because at Ezekial 4:11 we are instructed to drink each day "...water...by measure, the sixth part of a hin..." that computes to about 21 ounces per day.

I need about six glasses of fluids per day. I get most of that from coffee, tea, and food. If I do drink water, I drink pure water. I also use pure water for making my coffee, tea, and cooking. I buy bottled spring water. If I run out of that, I filter my tap water to remove the chlorine and fluoride.

The way chlorine got into your water is interesting. US factories were built to manufacture a lot of poison gas to kill our enemies during the two World Wars, I and II.

Peace brought with it its own problems though; one was what to do with all the leftover poison gas. It would cost a ton of money to "safely dispose" of it all. Yankee ingenuity gave us the answer: Let's put it in our drinking water. After all, it will kill all the bugs in the water, and this poison gas will make our drinking water safe...to...uh...drink...safe to drink.

So that is how chlorine got in our drinking water; our government put it there. So filter it out before you "drink the water." There are several good pitcher filters: Brita, PUR, etc. I use PUR and keep it in the ice box. Otherwise, buy spring water to avoid these poison gases including fluoride.

Twitter Profile

Fluoride is a poisonous byproduct of making aluminum. The aluminum manufacturers thought to themselves, *"If the government is stupid enough to buy chlorine, maybe they will be stupid enough to buy our waste product as well."* They thought right.

Even though: "Fluoride seems to fit in with lead, mercury, and other poisons that cause chemical brain drain," stated Philippe Grandjean, the adjunct professor of environmental health at the Harvard School of Public Health (HSPH). Cited from the article: Fluoride in private wells is linked to decreased IQ… found at http://www.naturalnews.com/046729_fluoride_private_wells_decreased_IQ.html#ixzz3COQoxvr1 (Accessed November 21, 2014) So filter out the fluoride as well.

Now about toothpaste: It is getting harder and harder to find toothpaste that doesn't have a fluoride additive. Tom's used to be a good one, but read the label. The best idea is to make your own toothpaste out of baking soda, Himalayan pink salt, and coconut oil. - More about salt and oil later when we talk about secondary foods. First the primary foods basics of exercise, water, and…sleep. We talked about exercise and water, next is sleep.

Tomorrow is another day…must rest…

"SLEEP IS THE BEST MEDITATION" – DALAI LAMA XIV

And "Meditation is the best treatment for insomnia."
–G. E. Frazier, CHC

Sounds like circular logic, but the point is this: Learn to meditate and sleep will come naturally.

1. "Why is sleep so important?" you ask.

Think of your brain as your body's organic hard drive. During your first four hours of sleep, your brain cleans itself. Spinal fluid washes through your brain, cleaning out the day's junk, technically called lectin. Memories are stored. Synapses are repaired and rewired. It is sort of...an extensive reboot.

The last four hours of sleep are spent in a spiritual place. It is a time and place to upload, download, and analyze data. This extraordinary place is called dreamland. (Lose your first four hours of sleep and lose your mind. Lose your last four hours of sleep and lose your soul.) I don't know whether it is true or not, but I've heard it said that "sociopaths do not dream." So, you see, you do need eight hours of sleep. Continuous and uninterrupted sleep is best, but try to maintain a consistent circadian cycle.

2. "How do I fall asleep in the first place?" you inquire.

One half hour before bed, eat one date and a handful of sunflower seeds. These two foods contain melatonin and will put you right to sleep. Balance that with some protein and fat, like you find in a half-a-glass of whole milk. If you use melatonin tablets, do so only occasionally, so as not to become dependent on them.

3. "What about muscle cramps?" you wonder.

I keep a bottle of potassium tablets on the nightstand beside my bed. Along with gentle stretching and massage, one tablet under my tongue relieves my charley horse. One tablet is enough. I don't overdo it; I remember that my heart is a muscle too.

4. "What if I wake up in the middle of the night?" you ponder.

If you wake up in the middle of the night, go back to bed ASAP. Even if you do not go back to "sleep," lying in bed will be restful for your body. However, meditate and you *will* go back to sleep. Consciously relax your muscles. Starting at your toes, relax each muscle, and move your attention to the next muscle until... *Whoops* ... It's morning. ...

5
Honor Your Ancestors

November 20, 2011, at 9:30 a.m.

And a glorious morn it is. Best night's sleep ever. I give thanks out loud, "Thanks be to...? Our ancestors." It is their genes that have evolved down to each of us.

This is one of our healing *principles: Be grateful* and express your appreciation. If you believe in an intelligent Creator, that's great. If you don't, you at least have to admit that our genes have been programmed, if not deliberately by design, then accidentally by...uh...by accident, to operate your body on the food that was available to your ancestors.

That is the basis for the Paleo Diet and the Ketogenic diet: Eat *what* your ancestors ate and *when* your ancestors ate. They were hunters and gatherers. They didn't hunt vegetables. They hunted animals.

Got your attention now?

There are some B vitamins that you get from eating animal products that you just don't get from any other source. Vitamin B12 is especially important for brain health. Sure you can take pills to supplement. But is that what you really want? To be dependent on manufactured synthetic vitamins?

About 20 percent of the population is Dawn Phenomenon and should not be vegetarian. About 50 percent of diabetics are Dawn Phenomenon and should not be vegetarian. Fifty percent? This calls for someone to investigate why. Could it possibly be an indication that 50 percent of diabetics are misdiagnosed? ... More on misdiagnosis later.

We are all concerned about the ethical treatment of animals. Therefore, buy your meat in the supermarket where no animals are ever harmed. ...And, join P.E.T.A., People Enjoying Tasty Animals.

Another question: When did our ancestors hunt animals?

At dawn.

~·~

Your ancestors survived long enough to procreate, so they were in the group that had the energy necessary at dawn to go out and hunt down their breakfast.

What did their genes tell their bodies to do to get ready for the morning hunt? Around 3:00 a.m., their genes, the precursors to your genes, told the liver and kidneys to begin producing glucose (sugar) and put it into the bloodstream, where it is immediately available for energy at dawn. (The circadian cycle at work...)

Their genes then kept their blood glucose levels high until some protein was eaten and detected in the bloodstream, thus signaling another successful breakfast.

"Eat breakfast, even if your blood sugar is high. Eating something will actually shut down the Dawn Phenomenon process and let your blood sugar return to normal."

Sources:

"The Dawn Phenomenon." DOC News. 01 Jul 2006. Volume 3 Number 7 p. 5 American Diabetes Association. 24 Nov 2007.

So, the ADA knew about the Dawn Phenomenon as early as 2006. Yet they kept quiet. Nary has a word been heard about the effect "the Dawn Phenomenon" has on the standard "fasting" blood glucose test results. Today, if you ask them about it, they will state that everyone is Dawn Phenomenon. It is no big deal. This is their way of minimizing it, so as not to face the questions that it raises. Inconsistencies in logic raise many questions about the basic nature of "type 2 diabetes." Questions about the efficacy of current medical practices: prevention, diagnosis, and treatment.

Your body functions the same today as did the body of any of your ancestors 6,000 years ago. Just as happened then, immediately after breakfast, your liver and kidneys stop producing glucose, and your pancreas starts producing insulin. Your insulin patrols your bloodstream looking for excess glucose and escorts it into your fat cells to be changed into fat and stored there (around your middle) until it is needed again for energy. Because your ancestor may not catch any food tomorrow, or the day after that, and stored fat will be necessary in order for him or her to survive. (The survival mechanism at work...)

Insulin's job is *not* to clear glucose out of your blood. That is merely a side effect of insulin's real role, which is to escort your glucose into your cells.

~·~

Don't all doctors know this?

No, they don't. When I asked Dr. Smith about the Dawn Phenomenon, he said, "What's that?"

This puts us, Dawn Phenomenon, in real danger of being misdiagnosed as diabetic and given dangerous Rx drugs that make us develop diabetes. (I'll tell you how in a moment. Pay attention because these drugs can cause harm to all patients not just to Dawn Phenomenon.)

It is not my doctor's fault. Doctors are not taught about the Dawn Phenomenon. They are taught that "sugar diabetes" was, prior to 1922, a problem with no solution.

Then, in 1922, Dr. Frederick Banting isolated what we now call insulin, which is the hormone that escorts sugar from the bloodstream into the cells. This was a tremendous discovery and benefit for those deficient in insulin from birth, (type I diabetes).

However, Doctors were surprised to find that some of their diabetic patients had plenty of insulin, yet still had high blood sugar. Well, they must be insulin resistant, the doctors reasoned, and type II diabetes was invented.

Giving insulin to those with type I helps those with type I, therefore, it was argued, giving more insulin to those with type II will help them too. And so it seemed… to help…helped the sales of insulin to increase, that is.

The only downside is that larger and larger doses of insulin are required to keep your blood sugar under control. Until finally your pancreas gives up and stops working altogether. And you do become a true diabetic, type I.

And that is how insulin shots cause diabetes.

Oh, and did I mention that insulin also makes you fat? This is in direct opposition to your goal of losing weight in order to control your blood sugar naturally.

But neither of these two side effects harms the drug companies, so Big Pharma has an incentive to incentivize the medical schools to keep on teaching future doctors to prescribe more and more insulin. It goes something like this:

"Well, we here at Medical Every State School (MESS) do appreciate the money we get from you drug manufacturers, but…"

"But what?" the drug manufacturers' representative demands.

"Well, it is just that most type II diabetics have higher than average insulin levels. It seems counterintuitive to give them more insulin. Why don't we try to find out *why* their cells are resisting the insulin and not taking on the glucose?" asks the MESS dean.

"Dean, you don't seem to understand. It is the revenue from the sales of insulin that makes it possible for us to help out medical schools like yours."

"Well, some of the new medical students here think that the cause may be something irritating the receptors on the cell walls. It may be diet related. If the fat cell's receptors swell from inflammation, the glucose may have trouble getting into the fat cells. And maybe we could prove that we need to reduce inflammation rather than increase insulin. If we can get some funding for those studies…"

"There will be no money for any such studies. Period," the drug manufacturers' rep responds emphatically.

"Well, if too much sugar in the blood is the problem, instead of giving more insulin, why not prescribe eating less sugar?" The dean states doggedly.

"Dean, you really do want to bite the hand that feeds you, don't you?"

The dean continues, "Well, I just…" Only to be cut off by the rep.

"You just…keep teaching what we tell you to teach. Sugar is sugar. Sugar is a carbohydrate. A carbohydrate is a carbohydrate. Carbohydrates give you calories. A calorie is a calorie. You know all this by looking at them under a microscope. There is no medical effect to eating one kind of calorie versus eating another kind of calorie. It is called the practice of medicine. Medicine is practiced by prescribing medicine…drugs. Drugs give us predictable, measurable results. Can you say that about diet changes?"

Not sure whether to agree with the rep or not, the dean has to admit, "Well, no."

"Why is it that medical schools don't waste time teaching nutrition?"

The medical school dean feels he must defend his school. "Well, I don't know. No studies have been done..."

Again he is cut off by the confident ranting of the drug manufacturers' rep: "It is part of the great divide between agriculture and medicine. We don't tell Big Agriculture how to engineer... I mean, how to farm food, and they don't tell us how to profit from... I mean, how to prescribe medicine. Our food is produced by those who know nothing about health, and our healthcare is provided by those who know nothing about food—and we aim to keep it that way. Don't we? It is called preserving the status quo."

The dean finally gives in, "Well, if you say so."

"We here at Every Drug Company's Lobby Group work for the drug manufacturers, and *they* say so."

~·~

The fasting blood glucose test

What is the standard medical procedure that your doctor follows in order to diagnose diabetes? He/she measures what they call your "fasting blood glucose." If it is over 110, you are diagnosed diabetic. Simple, right? Yes, too simple.

What is "fasting blood glucose"? According to your doctor, that is the amount of glucose (sugar) in your blood before breakfast, after your insulin has had all night to clear out the excess glucose in your blood and before you have eaten any sugar or other carbohydrate.

Those in the medical establishment have forgotten that your liver and kidneys produce glucose (sugar). They believe that you can only get glucose in your bloodstream by eating sugar, or other carbohydrates. You haven't eaten. You've been sleeping all night and haven't "broken fast" yet by eating breakfast (break-fast). They believe that before breakfast is when your blood glucose *should* be at its lowest point of the day, which *should* be a "normal" blood glucose reading of one hundred or less.

Under this official theory, your blood glucose level rises each and every time you eat. It goes higher and higher from the time you eat breakfast until two hours after your last bedtime snack. The time just before bedtime is *supposed* to be your highest blood glucose level of the day. Then, at night, your body's insulin begins to clear your bloodstream of any excess glucose (sugar). During the night your blood glucose level gets lower and lower until it reaches its lowest point just before breakfast.

It is under this false assumption that your doctor tells you not to eat anything before coming to his office, so he can take your "fasting blood glucose" reading. This is, to him, your lowest glucose level of the day.

But as we saw earlier, if you are a Dawn Phenomenon, then your glucose is high in the morning and stays high until you *do* eat breakfast. Then as you eat, your insulin begins to go to work storing your excess blood glucose as fat. And as a side effect, your insulin lowers your blood sugar during the day, and throughout the night, until reaching your lowest blood sugar level at 3:00 a.m.

What happens at 3:00 a.m.? The Dawn Phenomenon's healthy liver begins putting glucose into your bloodstream. Consequently, your blood glucose level begins rising from 3:00 a.m. until you *do* eat breakfast. This means that your highest blood glucose level is just before breakfast, just when your doctor thinks your blood glucose level should be at its lowest level.

See the problem?

To avoid this problem, be sure and ask for the "A1c test." Or better yet, order one yourself. No prescription is needed. You can purchase an A1c kit for around $50. A1c is an average of the glucose in your blood over the last three months. A1c works by measuring the blood glucose on your red blood cells. Red blood cells live for three months. So you end up with a measurement of your average glucose level for the last three months.

BTW, don't bother telling your doctor about the above. I tried. He just asked me whether or not I was depressed. See, if I don't tow the official line, I must be crazy and need antidepressant drugs.

BUT I HAVE PROOF

As you should too, I kept a journal. My blood glucose readings are higher in the morning before breakfast than they are the night before. I didn't eat during the night, so where did that glucose come from? Why didn't my insulin clear it out during the night, as the official theory states it will?

My actual blood glucose readings support the Dawn Phenomenon scenario. See for yourself on the following table:

Blood Glucose Readings for G. E. Frazier

DATE	"FASTING" READING BEFORE BREAKFAST	NIGHT TIME BEFORE BED
11/17/11	155 At doctor's office.	No Test Taken Tonight or tomorrow as I didn't get my monitor until 11/19/11.
11/19	169	157
11/20	176	142
11/21	173	210 - Souplantation!
11/22	175	127
11/25	166	138
11/26	140	116
11/28	155	110
11/29	172	111
11/30	161	134
12/1	Fly to Hawaii	---

POINT IS THAT MY "FASTING" READING IS CONSISTENTLY HIGHER THAN MY READING THE NIGHT BEFORE. EXCEPT FOR 11/21 WHEN I ATE A BIG MEAL LATE AT NIGHT AT SOUPLANTATION.

Source: G. E. Frazier's Journal

Normal is one hundred. So, at this point in time, my numbers are too high. And I am determined to reduce them. How I do that, and discover health, is my story. If you need to reduce your blood glucose numbers, what I did to reduce mine, will work for you too, whether or not you are Dawn Phenomenon.

At this point, 11/30/11, you could say that I am a diabetic Dawn Phenomenon. But I don't say that, because I don't believe that I am diabetic. And this mindset is very important to my recovery. I will not accept anything short of a full recovery. I believe with all my being that there is a cure. I am determined to find it. I will find it.

With my doctor's diagnosis of diabetes, I could apply for a handicap placket and park in the handicap spaces. I won't apply. I am not diabetic, and I am certainly not handicapped.

~·~

I am talking mainly to the approximately 20 percent of us who are Dawn Phenomenon. We are usually blood type O, personality type A, aggressive, determined, individualistic individuals. (And handsome too - even the women are handsome.) If you are not one of the 20 percent, be patient because I have answers for you, too. In the meantime, it is astute of you to have considered the possibility of being Dawn Phenomenon.

~·~

Why isn't everyone Dawn Phenomenon? Even though I believe that every healthy person is, or should be Dawn Phenomenon, Dr. D'Adamo provides another explanation:

A good discussion is found in the groundbreaking book, *Eat Right For Your Type* by Dr. D'Adamo. This book makes a compelling case that the answer is Darwin's Theory of Evolution within a species. Dr. D'Adamo believes that eighty percent of the human species learned how (evolved) to survive on wheat or other plant-based foods. This is in line with the *principle of biodiversity*: What is good for one is not necessarily good for another and certainly not good for all.

Coincidentally, this principle is why socialism doesn't work. What the glorious leader thinks is good for him/her, is not good for all, e.g., the first lady's school lunch dictates. I agree that school lunches need to be improved. And I applaud her efforts to bring attention to the school lunch problem and to educate the public. However, while her intentions are good and honorable, most decisions should not be made at the top, they should be made at the lowest level possible: Sometimes that means at the parental level. Sometimes individuals should be left to make their own decisions that affect them personally, especially when it comes to diet and health care decisions.

I say, "Especially diet and health care decisions," in line with another principle—that of *intuition*. You know your own body better than anyone. Trust your own body to know what to do to heal itself.

Did you know that the medical and dental professions are surprised to learn that your body can heal itself, even your teeth? Provided you let them. Just give your body exercise, hydration, good food, and sleep, all in harmony with your own body. These are the basics.

Some doctors are referring their "diabetic" patients to health coaches. This saves the doctor's time, as the doctor has only about seven minutes per patient. The health coach will devote forty-five to fifty minutes every two weeks to you. (In the beginning I want to see my "insulin resistant" clients once a week.) We have a lot to do so that your body can cure itself.

We must work with your medical doctor or other health care provider, especially if you are taking medicine, including insulin. Small changes in your diet and lifestyle can make such big changes in your body that your doctor may have to reduce your meds. We don't want your blood glucose level to drop too low.

First thing we do is to find out your specific health history, body type, what's been eating you, and what you've been eating.

Let's take a closer look at diet...

6
Standard American Diet (Sad)

November 21, 2011, at 9:00 a.m.

"The problem is we are not eating food any more, we are eating food-like products."
–Dr. Alejandro Junger

You are what you eat. And most of us eat the Standard American Diet, or SAD. That SAD stuff goes right into your blood. Your life is in your blood, and your blood is your life.

Ever since 1996, the year of the Kamikaze Cowboy diet disaster, I hadn't given much thought to food. In his book, *Confessions of a Kamikaze Cowboy: A True Story of Discovery, Acting, Health, Illness, Recovery, and Life*, Dirk Benedict relates how he cured himself of cancer with his diet. His diet worked for *him* to cure his cancer. Unfortunately, his diet did not help me to stay healthy, not that I didn't give his diet a good try.

I gave up all meat. I gave up all sugar, even fruit because fruit contains sugar. I gave up all spices. Dirk said to eat mostly grains and some vegetables. I followed the diet for one year, right up until In-N-Out came to San Diego.

That, and the fact that my saliva stopped digesting the grain. I ate grains: wheat, oats, and brown rice, for a year... raw. I would soak the grain overnight and then eat it raw the next morning. Naturally it took a lot of chewing before I could swallow it. After almost a year of this, I began to notice that the wheat grain would no longer liquefy, no matter how long I chewed. Instead, it turned into a gelatinous mass that refused to break up small enough to swallow. It's a good thing that I didn't swallow much of that, because I now know that what was left in my mouth, what I was trying ineffectively to chew and swallow, was... pure gluten. After a year of raw grains, my body changed the composition of my saliva to protect itself, me, from eating gluten.

Another *principle*: *Trust your body to know what is good for your body.*

And a good rule: Chew your food. Chewing is the beginning of the digestive process. For that reason I do not recommend juicing or smoothies. We need to chew our food. Juicing might be a good way to jump start your nutrition, but I do not recommend it for longer than a few weeks.

The raw-food diet is in this category too. Contrary to popular belief, our ancestors discovered fire rather early on. Cooking enhances most food. Tomatoes and kale are good examples. That said, low heat usually works best, and, for example, you only need to gently wilt your kale. And that takes no more than five minutes.

I went off that vegetarian diet in style though: one In-N-Out cheeseburger with fries and a chocolate ice cream milkshake.

I went home and threw it all up. True story.

~·~

Discouraged by that experience, I no longer tried to eat for health. I now ate instead for taste and convenience, which translates to mostly fast-foods, "Diners, Drive-Thrus, & Dives," as they say.

I always thought that the Souplantion, one of my favorite restaurants, was healthy: fresh produce to make your own salad followed by soups made daily from scratch. But take a look at my table, a few pages back, in chapter 5. When I took my glucose reading a few minutes after leaving this healthy establishment it was 210, the highest reading I had ever taken. What happened? Desserts happened, specifically, chocolate lava cake, soft-serve ice cream, and cookies. I would find out later that your blood sugar goes up as soon as you digest your food. It then takes two hours for your insulin to catch up and lower your blood glucose level by escorting that sugar into your cells to be turned into fat. That is why it helps to slow your digestion down—to give your insulin more time to do its job. You can slow down your digestion by taking cinnamon capsules and/or eating a lot of fiber.

So I take one gram of cinnamon before each meal. This slows my digestion down, giving my insulin time to do its job and also giving my intestines more time to absorb all of the nutrients from my food. I found some cinnamon capsules at Walmart and began taking about five grams per day. More about cinnamon later.

Fiber does the same thing. Eat green leafy vegetables, other vegetables, and fruits, depending upon your individual type.

Follow the *"eat variety" principle*: Consume the rainbow. Besides green, eat red apples, oranges, purple blueberries, etc.

Health coaches are trained to give you principles and broad rules to follow rather than specific foods and quantities. We trust you to listen to your body, to know, and to exercise your judgment. If left to your innate wisdom, you would choose nutrient-dense foods like the superfood, dark chocolate.

Health coaches help you figure out the *how*. You are busy. How are you going to find the time to fit in all the things you know you want to do? Ask your health coach.

Eating healthy is all in your mind. It is an attitude. Think of food as fuel for your body. And your body is a nice car. - A Mercedes. - You wouldn't fill a Mercedes with junk fuel. You wouldn't put sugar in your gas tank.

It is becoming a well-known fact that sugar is bad for you. Even the Simpsons had an episode chronicling the bad effects of sugar and its addictive nature. In the story, sugar pills were banned and replaced with "less addictive" opium pills. Sugar was banned, as well as anything containing sugar. Homer went to the supermarket and the shelves were empty, presumably because everything contains sugar. Homer and some others went to Mexico to smuggle in sugar. For a cartoon, that episode is very true to life.

~·~

"Sugar? What sugar? I didn't eat any candy today," you say.
 Okay, what did you eat?
 "French fries...with catsup"
 And to drink?
 "Pepsi."
 Anything else?
 "Lunch meat on Wonder Bread... Why are you looking at me like that? It's healthy. Scientists have added eight vitamins. ... Scientifically added. ...Vitamins. ...Eight."
 Principle: Question Authority. You should question even my statements and insights. I am giving you my opinions based upon my experiences. Hopefully you are finding some valuable gems that stand up to the fire of your inspection.

Standard American Diet (Sad)

First let's look at this Standard American Diet (SAD): French fries from white potatoes and white bread; both are loaded with starch. Three or more sugar molecules strung together makes one molecule of starch. That is why starch raises your blood glucose level faster than sugar and three or four times higher than sugar.

And that catsup is loaded with refined sugar too. Read the label.

The substitution principle: Now is the time to think substitution. Substitute sweet potatoes for white ones. Sweet potatoes actually lower blood glucose levels because they are full of fiber. Eat sprouted whole grain bread instead of white bread—again fiber versus no fiber. I buy Ezekiel 4:9 bread. Better yet, find, or make, wheatless bread with coconut flour.

Instead of catsup, put real butter, cinnamon, and pink salt on that sweet potato. If you need a little sweetener, add maple syrup grade B. And real whipped cream sweetened with stevia. Who said you had to sacrifice anyway? I like to add a few walnuts...and pecans.

Relatively minor changes over time can make a big difference in your overall health and wellness. That's what will make a big difference in your own body's ability to fight off, not only diabetes, but most other degenerative diseases, as well.

"Over time? How much time?" you question.

Poor health accumulates over time. It takes time to reverse it.

It takes twenty-one days to create a habit. After that you will continue in your new habit of healthy life style. You can do three weeks, can't you?

"Be careful not to compromise what you want most for what you want now."
–Andy Warhol

Good sugars are:
- stevia (not Truvia®),
- raw honey,
- coconut sugar, and
- maple syrup grade B.

Truvia is a sugar alcohol produced from genetically modified corn. I know you understand that Genetically Modified Organisms (GMOs) are destructive in many ways. No? You never heard of GMOs?

GMOs, also known as genetically engineered foods, or Frankinfoods, are financed by the Bill and Linda Gates Foundation with tax free money. When the scheme is completed Bill Gate's investment in Monsanto stock will skyrocket. That is the plan anyway. The chemical companies, principally Monsanto and Dow, have decided that they know better than nature how to design the genes of our plants. The genes of the corn used in the making of Truvia are spliced and diced to alter their basic makeup. GMO corn makes its own pesticide right inside each kernel of corn. When we eat the GMO corn we get to eat that new unnatural pesticide. No one knows what it will do to us and to our environment. One effect is that bugs grow immune to it and come back stronger than before, so that the farmers have to purchase more and more pesticide from Monsanto. Umm?

Sugar alcohols are found to be bad for your health too. So there are two strikes against Truvia. Ironically, the sugar alcohol in Truvia does make a good pesticide.

~·~

"Butter?"

Yes, real churned butter. Preferably from grass-fed pastured cows.

Dairy farmers and Dr. Mercola tell me that raw milk is healthy. And, it can help keep your gut supplied with healthy fauna and flora. This is especially so when you eat unsweetened yogurt, kefirs, and cheeses.

Many people cannot digest milk. I believe that is because the milk that you buy in the store is pasteurized. In fact, it is difficult to find raw milk.

Pasteurization is a process that heats raw milk to make the milk last longer. It kills bacteria and enzymes that are naturally in the milk and are needed by your body in order to digest that milk. Nature provides what your body needs and man destroys it. This is a clear example of the destruction of health by government under false pretenses. Big Dairy convinces people that healthy raw milk is unhealthy. And, supported by big media, gets it outlawed by your government.

Relative to diabetes: Unpasteurized milk contains cream that has enzymes that decrease insulin spikes and regulate the sugar absorption into your blood. Remember, the better your digestion the better your body will work. The less processing of your food (in other words, the closer to nature you can get your food), the better you will digest that food and all other food too.

The *whole food principle:* In the case of milk, that means all of the milk protein, sugar, and fat. Just the way it comes from the cow.

The *organic food principle:* Straight from the organic farmer is best. I am encouraged by the increase in the number of farmers' markets that I see.

~·~

Speaking of fat; if you don't want to be fat, eat more good fats, and eat a balance of saturated and unsaturated fats. We eat too

much vegetable oil, like corn oil. So eat more of the good fats, such as:
- wild game,
- wild fish,
- grass-fed meats and dairy,
- olive oil,
- coconut oil,
- walnuts,
- avocados, and
- flax seeds.

~·~

I haven't been feeling my best today. It is a good day to give this healthy eating a try. I decide to eat some broccoli—raw.

I wash it thoroughly. While it is draining, I get some mayo from the refrigerator. I put four tablespoons of it in a small bowl and season it. Let's see what I have in the cupboard: two teaspoons of minced garlic, several shakes of salt, and both black and red pepper. I hear that red pepper stimulates the pancreas to produce insulin. The salt is my special Himalayan pink salt with 30 percent less sodium and over eighty trace elements. I hear that northern sea salt is good too.

I cut my broccoli into bite-size pieces, giving thanks with a little prayer. Prayer is a type of meditation. I dip some dark-green broccoli into my fresh dip, chew it thoroughly… and a rush of energy rises from the approximate area of my feet, this wave of good feeling washes over me.

Is it the fact that the broccoli is raw, the oil in the mayo, the garlic, the red or black pepper, the minerals and trace elements in the pink salt, or this particular combination? Whatever it is, I like it.

I think it is my body appreciating that I am giving it something it needs. Whatever that something is, doesn't really matter.

Standard American Diet (Sad)

As I mentioned before, what matters is the *principle of variety*: One way to insure that your body gets what it needs is to eat a variety. One way to insure variety is to eat seasonally. In the summer nature gives us melons to cool us. In the winter we get oranges for vitamin C. It is best not to fool Mother Nature. Just accept the produce that is in season in your locale. (Seasonal produce is less expensive too.)

Wash it all down with a good seasonal red wine: merlot, Chianti, red table wine. As apostle Paul said in 1 Timothy 5:23, "Be no longer a drinker of water, but use a little wine for your stomach's sake and your own frequent infirmities." The key word here is "little." One or two glasses four or five times a week; and, remember the *principle of moderation in all things*.

~·~

I am learning that I should eat a balance of protein, oil, and carbohydrates. Forty percent of our calories should come from protein, 40 percent from fat and oil, and 20 percent from carbs. Volume wise, it works out to about equal portions of each, since carbs take up more space on your plate than do oils or protein.

This could be rather boring except for the wonderful world of herbs and spices. In general herbs and spices stimulate your digestive system, which helps you metabolize your food.

Spices, such as like cinnamon, cayenne, turmeric, cumin, are all helpful for keeping you humming along like a well-oiled machine. In fact the top six herbs and spices for weight loss are:

1. Cinnamon—boosts metabolism, helps maintain healthy weight, regulates blood sugar. The metabolism of glucose is increased by about 20 percent when cinnamon is consumed. Reduces triglycerides, LDL (bad cholesterol),

and total cholesterol. More on cinnamon later. The main thing is that cinnamon makes your coffee sexier and healthier.

2. Turmeric—contains curcumin, which suppresses blood vessels necessary to form fat tissue, may lower both body fat and weight gain.

3. Cumin—produces energy and aids in digestion. It provides glycemic control, is an antistressor, and improves memory.

4. Ginger—relaxes and sooths the intestine. It is anti-inflammatory, boosts metabolism and suppresses appetite.

5. Dandelions—every part is edible. Contains antioxidants, bitter crystalline compounds: taracerin, inulin, taraxacin, and levulin. They also contain fiber, beta-carotene, and K1, plus other vitamins and minerals.

6. Mustard seeds—three-fifths teaspoon per day burns forty-five more calories per hour. It boosts metabolic rate by 25 percent.

7. And as a bonus, see also lion's mane mushrooms.

This list is not all inclusive by any means. There are many other good ones as well. Sources for more information are:
http://dailyhealthpost.com/15-herbs-spices-that-help-you-lose-weight/

Standard American Diet (SAD)

http://www.realfarmacy.com
http://www.stylecraze.com

~·~

Don't forget: eat more good fats and oils. Some vitamins are water soluble, some are oil soluble. It is the same with hormones. You cannot live without oils and fats. Your skin is mostly fat. Skin is the largest organ of your body. You want glowing healthy skin don't you?

If you are worried about bad cholesterol (LDL), the cinnamon you may be taking for blood-sugar control, will control your bad cholesterol too—and do so better than statin drugs, IMO.

Every country has their herbs and spices. Many are helpful for health and are worthy of study, especially, but not limited to:
- Chinese herbs and
- Indian herbs

There are several good books on herbs. I rely upon reference books. As I say, "My brain is on my bookshelf." When necessary, I can look it up.

Or, I can ask the Universal Mind; As I will explain in the next chapter ...

PART II
DECEMBER 2011

7
Primary Foods

December 1, 2011, at 4:45 a.m.

"To make the right choices in life you have to get in touch with your soul; to do this you need solitude, which most people are afraid of, because in the silence you hear the truth and know the solutions."
–Deepak Chopra

You can get in touch with your soul every night during sleep. Ask the burning questions, and then sleep on it. Write the solutions down before you get up, while you are yet half awake, in that space between sleep and alertness. You are still slipping in and out between this world and that world, the world of dreams - even groggy. "Grog" is the old English word for rum. As you slowly sober up from the morning's grogginess, the answer is there. It has been there all along, but now you see it clearly. And you know intuitively that it is the only answer that makes sense. Some practice this every morning and call it "morning pages."

Now spring to your feet and into action.

Ha. Easier said than done.

What time is it? I ask myself.

Some unintelligible chatter is coming through my alarm clock radio. I stretch my neck sideways, looking to my clock radio for the answer to my question. The LED lights glare 4:45.

Four forty-five a.m.? Why so early? ... Then it dawns on me.

Oh, today I fly to Hawaii. I had better get up.

Fifteen pushups and a shower and I am ready. My friend Lupe gives me a ride to the airport. And I am off for fun and sun in paradise.

This is *the principle of R and R: relaxation and rewarding* yourself with the rewards of the primary foods of relationships and family ties. I am going to see my son and daughter-in-law and two grandsons. They live in Hawaii.

Diet and food are secondary foods. Of first importance are primary foods. If you are not balanced in the primary foods, you are not going to be healthy, no matter how healthy the food on your plate.

There are twelve primary "foods." I will list them here because, "Even a dull pen is better than a bright memory."

1. Career
2. Education
3. Confidence
4. Spirituality
5. Creativity
6. Social Life
7. Home environment
8. Home cooking
9. Finances
10. Health
11. Physical activity
12. Relationships

For further study on the vital topic of primary foods, I recommend Joshua Rosenthal's book *Primary Foods*.

So I am off to renew and strengthen my relationships. Everything is intertwined. My son has a lot of outdoor physical-activities planned for us. My grandsons teach me creativity with their new tablets; iPads I believe they call them. I discover coconuts. The entire experience is very spiritual. But not paradise:

~·~

Not Paradise

"Was it the sweet smell of exotic blossoms wafting on the back of a river of humid air drifting in through the open windows?

Could-a-been the soft showers of warm neolani, dew from heaven, that pass by as regular as the marching bands in a well-orchestrated parade.

Must-a-been the unfamiliar songs of unknown birds whistling melodic greetings to the arrival of light peeking through cloud streaked skies.

The timelessness of now enfolds me, holds me in the midst of this mist of tropical air, warm upon my newly tanned face. I smile.

This is Not Paradise.
Just a dress rehearsal."

- G. E. Frazier

~·~

DECEMBER 2, 2011

At 4:30 a.m. I'm up and doing twenty push-ups. After breakfast we walk up a ridge to one of many pill boxes that were built during World War II. It is a terrific view of the island of Oahu. It is also a lot of exercise and sunshine.

Tonight we go to see the *Muppet Movie*. I eat too much popcorn. Then get my highest blood glucose reading ever: 214. From this experience I learn that starch from popcorn spikes your blood glucose.

DECEMBER 3, 2011

At 6:00 a.m. the next morning, I'm up and doing twenty-two push-ups. I go for a walk. When I get back, I take my blood glucose reading: 121.

We go snorkeling.

DECEMBER 4, 2011

At 7:30 a.m. I'm up and doing twenty-five push-ups. We go paddling one mile off shore into the Pacific Ocean, out to the Mokes…and one mile back.

DECEMBER 6, 2011

At 8:00 a.m. I'm up and doing thirty push-ups. We hike to the top of Diamond Head, an extinct volcano. There is an extensive pill box compound at the top. We explore it thoroughly. At the bottom of this mountain is a farmers' market where I find an assortment of treats. I buy a date bar. It contains organic dates, chocolate, almonds and other good stuff, but no processed sugar. It is very sweet, and the best part: eating it doesn't raise my glucose level. So I don't have to give up all of life's pleasures after all.

DECEMBER 9, 2011

At 9:00 a.m. I'm up and doing thirty-five push-ups. I discover fresh coconut; and my glucose readings drop to an acceptable level of 105. I think that eating the coconut helped lower my blood glucose level. Coconuts contain potassium, omega 3, lots of good protein, and fiber. They are fresh, in season, local, and organic. I stop and eat one at every roadside stand... of which there are many dozens.

Coconuts also contain L-Arginine, which activates the chicken pox retrovirus in my system. I don't know it yet, but when I get back home on December 17, I will get shingles: a painful lesson to teach me moderation in all things, including coconuts. And that's the truth. But then as Pontius Pilate famously said...

8
"What is Truth?" – Pontius Pilate in John 18:38

December 17, 2011, at 9:00 a.m.

Welcome home. There is no gas for cooking or for hot water. So I go to In-N-Out for a burger and to the gym for a shower. My left side is sensitive to the touch and to cold. The shower at the gym is cold... The cold water hits my back..."OUCH..." It is definitely shingles.

When I get back from the gym, I take Acidophilus, L-Lysine, echinacea, and vitamin C. I begin putting tea tree oil on the area. I don't know if it will help, but it can't hurt. Tea tree oil kills bacteria, fungus, and virus.

Principle: First do no harm, but it is okay to experiment... carefully...on yourself.

You noticed the In-N-Out burger didn't you? Apropos here as this is the truth chapter. But you see, today is Saturday. And Saturday is my weekly cheat day. On my cheat day I can eat anything I want, even margaritas with my friend Sebastian later today. One day a week, you must reset your metabolism in order to keep your body from going into starvation mode. Starvation mode is a survival mode. Your body senses that food has been rather sparse lately, so your body thinks there may be a famine. To prepare for less food being available, your body thinks for itself: *Better slow down the ol' metabolism and store the fat rather than burning it.*

Therefore, the cheat day; the cheat day lets your body know that all is well in the food availability department.

There is an alternative to having a cheat day: Eat reasonable meals all week and then have one starvation day per week.

As your health coach, I present alternatives to you at the proper moment. You choose the ones you like, and the ones that fit *you*. Together we design a plan best for *your* body type and lifestyle. Finally, I hold you accountable to your plan for wellness.

I do not practice medicine, I coach you to wellness.

Wellness is more of an art than a science. Science has lost its way. I do not rely on science, and here is why: Beginning in the 1950s, science became institutionalized. And with government and private money, science (including medical science) became elitist and arrogant and greedy for more money. The following is what the top historian of science has to say about truth, the people, control of science, and therefore the control of "truth":

Truth can be determined only by the judgment of experts... Everything is decided by very small groups of men, in fact, by single experts whose results are carefully checked, however, by a few others. The people have nothing to say but simply to accept the decisions handed out to them. Scientific activities are controlled by universities, academies and scientific societies, but such control is as far removed from popular control as it possibly could be.

–George Sarton, historian of science [Sarton (1955) P.12]

Science, Religion and Power by Rupert Sheldrake, I St. John..,
http://stjohnoneone.com/2013/03/01science-religion-and-power-by-rupert-sheldrake/ (accessed December 30, 2014)
Near the bottom of the web site
(also at footnote #9)

~·~

At www.SpaceDoc.Com you can find Dr. Graveline, a medical doctor and a former NASA astronaut. He and a whole host of doctors now warn against taking statin drugs like Lipitor and Crestor, two of the most popular cholesterol lowering drugs. Dr. Graveline admits to being so gullible that he never ate an egg for seventeen years. Now he believes that cholesterol is the most important biochemical in our body and has nothing to do with cardiovascular disease.

> ...We all listened to what amounts to brainwashing. The brainwashing that we got from 1955 on, to just recently... They have liberalized the diet stuff recently though, so people are back to eating eggs and drinking whole milk and eating butter. I went around recommending margarine for so long, and margarine is what's causing disease-butter is what's helping to cure it. It's incredible!
> —Dr. Duane Graveline

Lipitor: The Common Drug that Destroys Your Memory [or, Dr. Duane Graveline on Cholesterol and Coenzyme Q10 (CoQ10)] http://articles.mercola.com/sites/articles/archive/2011/02/12/dr-duane-graveline-on-cholesterol-and-coq10.aspx (Accessed November 30, 2014).

And who were the beneficiaries of all this brainwashing?... Big Pharma, such as AstraZeneca, the marketer of the drug

Crestor, the statin drug that is heavily advertised on TV today: - "Are you down with Crestor?" - Whatever that means...

Also benefiting were the makers of margarine: "I can't believe it's not butter." I can't believe we gave up wonderful butter so easily.

~·~

"This, of course, is nothing more than "mob science" which isn't really science at all. If new science were only recognized once all the existing scientists were convinced of its truth, then science would never have advanced."- Mike Adams (aka the "Health Ranger") is the founding editor of NaturalNews.com, the internet's No. 1 natural health news website, now reaching 7 million unique readers a month.

In late 2013, Adams launched the Natural News Forensic Food Lab, where he conducts atomic spectroscopy research into food contaminants using high-end ICP-MS instrumentation. With this research, Adams has made numerous food safety breakthroughs such as revealing rice protein products imported from Asia to be contaminated with toxic heavy metals like lead, cadmium and tungsten. Adams was the first food science researcher to document high levels of tungsten in superfoods. He also discovered over 11 ppm lead in imported mangosteen powder, and led an industry-wide voluntary agreement to limit heavy metals in rice protein products to low levels by July 1, 2015.

In addition to his lab work, Adams is also the (non-paid) executive director of the non-profit Consumer Wellness Center (CWC), an organization that redirects 100% of its donations receipts to grant programs that teach children and women how to grow their own food or vastly improve their nutrition.

"What is Truth?" – Pontius Pilate in John 18:38

Learn more: http://www.naturalnews.com/042112_TED_conferences_pseudoscience_GMO.html#ixzz3NRquZh68http://www.naturalnews.com/042112_TED_conferences_pseudoscience_GMO.html#ixzz3lneB0OLg/ (Accessed November 30, 2014).

Maybe science (including medical science) has not advanced in a long time! And that is one of the main points of this book.

~·~

Back to my confessions and more truth: In light of the fact that I do not believe in the safety of most Rx drugs, and in the spirit of full disclosure, I must tell you that today ... I begin daily dosing with Andro-gel, testosterone. Well, that guy in the TV commercial said I may have "Low T" ... and he looked so happy and energetic. I just had to try it.

My blood glucose readings are already quite low—take today for instance: 112.

That said, the effects of testosterone supplementation are nothing short of amazing. Now instead of dragging myself to the gym, I can't wait to begin my exercises. Instead of walking, I am running up stairs. I am getting admiring looks from young women. I have never had a "six pack" before. My mind is clearer. I am getting more done during the day...and during the night, if you get my drift.

But I would not do it again. That's because the list of side effects is long. Within two months, I notice that my feet and ankles are swelling. So I cut my dosage in half. When they are still swollen, I stop taking *T* altogether. I definitely do not want to become dependent on a Rx drug. On the other hand, I have no doubt that my increased metabolism due to the *T* has been helpful in reducing my blood glucose level.

~·~

"Where did Frazier go?" I hear in a booming voice. It's my friend Sebastian, a retired medical doctor. He is greeting me from across the parking lot. He cannot believe the transformation I have made to a slim trim 192 pounds.

He is impressed and wants to lose his extra pounds too.

Healthy lifestyle certainly has helped me reduce my weight and waist size. I went from 245 pounds and forty-five inches to 192 pounds and thirty-six inches, respectfully. That's right. I lost fifty-three pounds and nine inches around my waist in two months.

All I did was eliminate processed sugar and chemical sugar substitutes. I also reduced starches, such as white potatoes and white rice. I increased my consumption of Himalayan pink salt and good fats and oils, including butter. I get more exercise now, and I get ions; more on ions later. And I get lots of sunshine for the needed sunshine hormone "vitamin" D.

Sebastian and I are going to have a drink after work. We are both retired but not resigned. We both work when we feel like it.

~·~

I am sitting at the bar with Sebastian when I notice two men sitting directly across from us. I nudge Sebastian. "See those two old drunks across the bar? That's us in twenty more years."

Sebastian corrects me: "There are no two old drunks across the bar. That's a mirror."

We both agree to go easy on the margaritas and begin discussing hormone "vitamin" D.

~·~

Some time ago a scientist noticed that something, he didn't know what, was helping calcium to enter the bones. He reasoned that

"What is Truth?" – Pontius Pilate in John 18:38

it must be a vitamin. What to name it? Vitamins had recently been discovered, and the names were going fast. There were already vitamins A, B, and C. So...he named it...vitamin D.

This is an example of "one fatal flaw." One seemingly small error in language sets in motion a tiny error in thought, which, like the butterfly effect, results in unintended consequences.

This is the reason why we must insist upon the truth, no matter how small the matter seems or how hard the insistence upon it appears to be. Trust but verify; request reasonable proof. If the media had insisted on reasonable proof when Obama lied about ObamaCare, it would have never passed, and we would have saved trillions of dollars and millions of jobs. Imagine the health and wellness advancements that could have been made; if that money had been spent on real scientific study, instead of on increasing the size of government and on health insurance premiums.

But then what is truth? Is it what scientists say it is? Is it what the government says it is? Or is it what *you* experience and what you learn intuitively from the Universal Mind? To be truly free, you must be free to act in accordance with that which you know to be true. The only limit on your freedom should be a prohibition against you hurting others. Your right to swing your fist stops at my nose.

But, I digress. But, not really, as an author, I am supposed to use words in the same way as other people use them. That is called "exact diction." Readers expect the denotation of a word to be its exact literal "established meaning." (No wonder things are in such a mess. It seems as though you are not allowed to tell the truth until it is "established truth." How in the world do errors ever get corrected then?)

So dear editor, when I write *hormone* D, just think hormone "vitamin" D, if it makes you feel better.

Why do I say hormone D, instead of vitamin D? Let me explain...

9
Hormone D

December 17, 2011, at 5:30 p.m.

It is said that there is an epidemic of vitamin D deficiency. It isn't true, because there is no such thing as *"vitamin"* D. *Hormone* D begins with the sun. Sunshine on your bare skin starts the protocol whereby your body makes your own hormone D. The circuitous route by which your body makes its own hormone D is nothing short of miraculous.

First, the sun's rays, filtered through the earth's atmosphere, beam upon your bare skin. Next, your skin is warmed by these rays to produce perspiration. The sun's rays interact with your perspiration. Next, your perspiration is reabsorbed by your skin to make its way to your liver where it is hydroxylated into 25-hydroxy D. This is the major circulating form of hormone D, but it is still inactive. It first has to go to your kidneys to be modified again to its active form, 125-dihydroxy hormone D. Now it can do its hormonal work of telling your intestines to absorb calcium from your green vegetables. The green vegetables you eat every day. If you don't, you will now…won't you?

BTW, you do not get usable calcium from milk. You get calcium from the same place that cows get theirs—from green vegetables. Late-breaking news: Calcium supplementation is harmful to your heart and harmful to your teeth and bones too. But that is another book. Back to hormone D.

Hormone D is one of, if not the most, powerful gene activator in human biology, turning on "healing genes" like microscopic light switches.

I say hormone D rather than vitamin D, because 125-dihydroxy fits the definition of a hormone: a substance produced by one organ that goes into the blood to communicate with, and have an effect on, one or more other organs.

Upward of 40–60 percent of people are at risk for hormone D deficiencies. Seventeen percent more of you are hormone D deficient all year long due to wearing sunblock continuously.

Hormone D is important at birth to help prevent type I diabetes. And yet 81 percent of newborn babies are hormone D deficient at birth. Maybe we should give newborn babies hormone D instead of MMR vaccines that many believe can cause autism. But that is another topic for another day.

Warning: do not buy vitamin D at the store, as it is probably synthetic D2, which does more harm than good. Pills called vitamin D2 are worse than nothing.

Hormone D in the form of 125-dihydroxy can only be purchased with a doctor's prescription. But why waste your money, when nature gives you hormone D for free from the sun? You make hormone D by using the sun intelligently. You are the combination of your mind, your body, and your spirit. Decide to use the sun intelligently to gain from it the many benefits it offers your body and, ultimately nourishes your spirit.

Cancer from the sun?

There is more cancer in the Northern Hemisphere than there is at the equator.

Hormone D regulates cell growth and thereby prevents cancer.

Hormone D

The sunblock industry is big business. They promote the information that will sell more sunscreen. And they suppress information such as the following: In one study sunscreen reduced hormone D production by 95 percent. Sorry, I cannot give you a citation for this information as it has been successfully suppressed.

Forget sunscreen. Wear a hat. And ingest natural sun protection such as:
- astaxanthin,
- acai,
- pomegranates, and
- blueberries.

These protect you naturally from the sun's powerful rays. However, use your common sense in your sun exposure.

The American Academy of Dermatology is well funded by the sunscreen industry. The Safe Skin Association, funded by Coppertone, actually puts out paid news releases attacking anyone who says sunshine is good for you.

Again, think back to our ancestors: Our human species evolved in sunlight. We need five to thirty minutes of sun at least three times per week, depending on many factors. Dr. Michael Holick has a table in his book, *The UV Advantage*. Use this table. Time yourself. In order to avoid sunburn, don't stay in the sun more than your body type can handle.

If you do get sunburned, soak the area with apple cider vinegar.

Generally, thirty minutes outside in a bathing suit equals 20,000 international units (IU) of hormone D. So why pay for capsules that contain only 400 to 1,000 units?

Hormone D is good for brain development. We know that there is more depression on gloomy days; now we know why. Dr. Holick gives 50,000 IU of hormone D to treat depression.

Sunshine actually helps achiness in bones often diagnosed as fibromyalgia. Sunshine can reverse that. It'll take up to a year though.

Relative to diabetes: Hormone D regulates insulin secretion by your pancreas and increases insulin sensitivity.

Eighty-one percent of babies are hormone D deficient at birth, putting them at high risk of developing type I diabetes. Hormone D is very important in the first two years of life.

I was born in winter. My mother had the intuition to know that sunshine and fresh air would be good for me. So she put me outside around noon time in the snow. It was winter after all. Consequently I grew up strong and well suited for cold weather. The sun must have given me enough hormone D to build strong bones, because I have never had a broken bone in my entire life. That is so even though I have had many bumps and bruises in my life. Just the other night I stepped out of bed to go to the bathroom, forgetting that I was sleeping on the top bunk. Yep, I fell five feet onto the ceramic tile floor below. My seventy-year-old bones suffered no ill effects. Too bad we can't say the same for the floor.

In my search for health, I learned, not only about the need for hormone D from sunshine, but also about the need for ions. Ions also come from the sun. ...

And we can benefit from them by "earthing." ...

10
Earthing

December 18, 2011

Ions are molecules that have gained or lost an electrical charge. You may have experienced the power of negative ions when you set foot on the beach. Ions are created in many ways. The ones we are concerned with here are the strong ones that come from the sun. If they weren't screened out by the ionosphere, we would burn up. But our Designer also knew that we humans need ions in just the right amount to give us electrical energy and protection from inflammation.

So ions are delivered to us by way of lightning from the ionosphere to the earth's surface. We pick up ions through the bottoms of our feet. That is we used to, until we humans invented shoes.

I had another health advantage growing up. My parents couldn't afford to buy me shoes, so I went barefoot until I was seven years old. We lived across the street from a large park. I would roam that park, sometimes all day … getting hormone D, ions, and a tan you would not believe.

Nowadays, as part of my health regimen, I use a similar technique. To save time, I combine sunshine, exercise, fresh air, and ions in one activity: going to the beach.

So today I go to the beach.

I wear my cargo shorts and nothing else. I walk on the wet sand between the waves and the dry sand. Since ions are electrical, I figure the wetness of the wet sand will help transmit the ions into my feet.

I walk a mile and then turn around and walk back, for a total of two miles.

Today I see ahead of me a pretty girl doing the same thing as I am.

When I catch up to her, I introduce myself. "Hello. My name is Frazier. Are you earthing?"

She is barefoot but otherwise covered in loose white clothing and sporting a large floppy-brimmed white hat, which is smart because she has a very light complexion.

"Oh, hi. My name is Betty, and…why yes, I *am* earthing. … You too?"

"Yes. It is good exercise, fresh air, 'vitamin' D, and ions. Ions fight inflammation. And inflammation is implicated in every disease. So ions are very healthy. …Do you earth often?"

"No. I live twenty-five miles from the beach, so I don't get here very often. … It is nice to talk to someone while walking. … Have you read any good books lately?"

"As a matter of fact, I have finally gotten around to reading *Atlas Shrugged.*"

"Oh, I have read that two times." She allows herself to brag a little.

"Wow. I am impressed."

I notice a bee on the sand in front of us and call out a warning.

"Uh oh, watch out for that bee. You don't want to step on him. He will string your bare foot."

(As a warning to you: earthing is wonderful, but watch where you step.)

And on and on, we discover that we have more in common than earthing.

This is a side benefit, a primary food, that of socializing, sharing ideas, and empathizing with others. This is a very healthy practice.

So try earthing every other day. Even on the cold nippy days of winter. I've been earthing alone, on cold days that I could not find a friend, ... on blustery days when the wind, Mariah, blows empty trash bags across the grass, like so many plastic tumbleweeds.

Walking alone has its benefits too: communing with nature, meditating, thinking. It was Andy Warhol who said, "One is company, two is a crowd, and three or more is a party."

So when I walk alone, I think: *When fat comes out of your cells, it comes out as free fatty acids (FFA)s. Could it be FFAs, that are clogging up the works? And if we could get FFAs balanced with niacin, would diabetes be cured?*

When I walk alone I also think: *Could it be that insulin resistance is due to inflammation of the glucose receptors located in the cell walls? If insulin cannot usher glucose into the cells to be turned into fat, then insulin is unable to do its job. Could reducing inflammation be the key to curing diabetes? If so, then reducing inflammation by earthing will definitely help to cure diabetes.*

Sometimes I think: *Chlorophyll is a green crystal that is produced in plants when they receive sunlight. When you eat green vegetables, you are eating chlorophyll crystals made by the sun. These crystals enter your body and become your hemoglobin. Just another way that the Creator's sun gives us life, from the sun to our blood, and your life is in your blood. Chlorophyll crystals deliver magnesium where it is needed and remove heavy metals from our blood. Pretty amazing, and no one knows how this works. Gee, there is a lot of work to be done and discoveries to be made.*

I also think about the role of good fats and oils in your body. There are many oil-soluble functions in your body. You need to eat good fats and good oils. To lose your belly fat, eat more good fat.

Eat grass-fed animals, avocados, walnuts, flax seed, coconut oil, olive oil, and butter from grass-fed cows. Raw milk has many health enhancing properties. Raw milk has in it the enzymes needed to digest it. Yep, nature provided a complete package. It is man who destroyed the good enzymes and good bacteria by heating the milk (pasteurization) to make it last longer. Raw milk will last two to three weeks if you keep it cold.

And as with most things, moderation is the key.

Another *principle: variety, balance, and moderation.* As you may recall, I found this out with my over indulgence in coconuts. Sometimes you have to learn about life the hard way. And sometimes life is not fair. Such as when Miley Cyrus gets naked and licks a hammer, it is called art. When I do it, I have to put my clothes back on and leave Home Depot?

Interestingly, just last night, even *South Park* suggested that we should eat mostly fats and oils. So it is becoming well known that the sixty-year fad of eating low-fat and nonfat "foods" has been detrimental to our health.

Along with the health-and-wellness revolution, we are discovering good fats and oils, especially coconut oil...

11
Coconut Oil

December 19, 2011

There are no "bad" fats. There are three types of fats: short chain, medium chain, and long chain. Our bodies need all three types. Presently, Big Agriculture gives us almost exclusively the long-chain fat (corn oil). This puts us out of balance, so that we need more short-chain fats (olive oil). Therefore we call short-chain fats the "good" fats. Medium-chain oil is also a good fat. The most economical one is coconut oil. It has properties different than the other two.

Coconut oil has healthy properties both internally and externally. It is good for your tummy and for your skin.

Coconut oil stands up well to heat and is, therefore, suitable for cooking without burning. Also use it to heal or just to smooth your skin.

Unrefined extra virgin coconut oil contains lauric acid, which has powerful anti-microbial, anti-viral, and anti-fungal properties.

Perfect for the exciting, beneficial, healthy practice of…oil pulling.

According to paleoburn.com/coconuts-oil-pulling for the last 3,000 years, Ayurvedic literature has taught the use of oil pulling for improving oral, as well as systemic health. Oil pulling, or *Kavala*, has also been successfully used in the treatment of headaches, migraines, diabetes mellitus, asthma, and acne.

Oil pulling is quite simple. First thing in the morning, take about a teaspoon to a tablespoon of the coconut oil into your mouth and swish it around for approximately fifteen to twenty minutes.

You can start at ten minutes and work your way up to twenty minutes of swishing to clean out plaque and other bacteria. More than twenty minutes would be over swishing. You don't want the bacteria to re-enter your mouth, defeating the purpose of oil pulling.

Do *not* swallow the oil; it is inundated with the very bacteria and toxins you want to rid yourself of.

Do *not* spit the oil down the sink or flush it down the commode. Since coconut oil is solid at room temperature, it could build up in your home's pipes and plug up the plumbing.

This is according to Bruce Fife, CN, ND, a certified nutritionist and naturopathic physician. He is the author of twenty books, including *Coconut Cures and Oil Pulling Therapy: Detoxifying and Healing the Body through Oral Cleansing*. See more at www.grotonwellness.com/sites/default/files/DentalHealthOilSwishing.pdf.

Recent anecdotal evidence from loyal "pullers" has shown oil pulling to, among other things:
- strengthen teeth, gums, and jaws;
- prevent and treat oral diseases, such as gingivitis;
- prevent cavities;
- prevent bad breath;
- reduce gum bleeding; and
- prevent throat, mouth, and lip dryness.

One more anecdotal incident: About two weeks after I began oil pulling, I noticed an irritation in the back of my throat. I felt with my tongue a small bump at that spot. A few days later, I coughed up a very small amount of blood. A few days after that, and immediately after I finished my morning oil pulling, two small tumors (for lack of a better word) came out of the back of my throat. I spit them out, and, next, thick red blood flowed slowly, actually spreading like only blood can spread, from my left nostril. This small puddle of blood oozed down my upper lip, stopping just short of my mouth. The bump in the back of my throat disappeared. I knew right then and there that my body had just healed itself from whatever...with the help of the coconut oil.

The list of amazing benefits should be enough to interest you in giving oil pulling a try. There have never been any documented negative side effects.

You didn't know oil was so good for you, did you? Where else have we been misled? What other healthy things have we been denied all in the name of good health?

Let's pull back the curtain. And look at L-GAAT, (Lies - Generally Accepted As True)...

12
A Partial List of L-GAAT, Lies - Generally Accepted as True

December 20, 2011

"It ain't what you don't know that gets you into trouble. It's what you know for sure that just ain't so."
–Mark Twain

Much is made of GAAT, or knowledge Generally Accepted As True. Well let's look at what society, and possibly you yourself, "know for sure that just ain't so."

L-GAAT, Lies - Generally Accepted As True. These are untruths that most people accept as true. Let's list the lies we've already run into.

- Poor health does NOT cause disease. Disease is caused by a deficiency of pharmaceutical drugs in your body.
- Diabetes is incurable.
- Diabetes is caused by too much sugar in your blood.
- Insulin's main job is to clear sugar out of your blood.

- You need more insulin, regardless of how much insulin you do or don't already have.
- Cinnamon does nothing one way or another for anything, especially not for diabetes.
- Flu shots keep you from having the flu.
- Flu shots can't possibly hurt you.
- MMR vaccinations are safe.
- Sugar is good for you. It's the real thing.
- Sugar makes you happy. Well, this one is true…in the short run. However, it is untrue in the long run. We have much to learn about sugar and how it is just as addicting as cocaine.
- Sugar is not a poison.
- Diabetes Rx drugs keep your diabetes from getting worse.
- The government will protect you. You don't have to take personal responsibility for your own health.
- The Affordable Care Act is affordable.
- The Affordable Care Act will add no new taxes.
- The Affordable Care Act will result in the average family saving $2,500 per year on insurance premiums.
- If you like your insurance, you can keep your insurance.
- If you like your doctor, you can keep your doctor.
- Government cares about my health.
- Don't expect to live healthy to age 120.
- It is impossible to control diabetes with diet and exercise.
- Rx drugs will control your diabetes so that you can safely continue your unhealthy life style.
- It is good to add the poisons chlorine and fluoride to your water.
- No one needs meat. Everyone should be vegetarian.
- Fasting blood glucose level is the day's lowest level for everyone.

A Partial List of L-GAAT, Lies - Generally Accepted as True

- Medical schools can accept money from Big Pharma and remain independent.
- Doctors can accept money from Big Pharma and remain independent.
- Government can accept money from Big Pharma and remain independent and independently regulate Big Pharma to protect us, the consumers of health care.
- Medical researchers can accept money from Big Pharma and remain independent.
- Big Media can accept money from Big Pharma and remain independent.
- We consumers are not being sold Rx drugs in the same way that we are sold sugary soft drinks and beer.
- If you don't tow the official line, you must be crazy.
- That big government knows what is best for us, so we should accept ObamaCare. Just like Wonder Bread and margarine, it's based on science. And remember what science thinks of us. Their view of the general public was recently confirmed by this late-breaking news: Professor Jonathan Gruber, the head architect of ObamaCare, was caught on tape confirming our worst fears. It seems that videotape has surfaced of him stating that it was necessary to lie about ObamaCare in order to pass it, and we, the people, are too stupid to know that we are being lied to.
- Your body cannot heal itself; in order to heal, your body must have drugs and surgery.
- Wheat and other grains should be the staples of your diet.
- Fats and oils should be eliminated from your diet.
- Salt should be eliminated from your diet.
- Milk must be pasteurized.
- Processed food is good for you.

- Fat makes you fat.
- Lose weight by eating less and exercising more.
- A calorie is a calorie is a calorie.
- Starch does not raise your glucose level.
- Diet sodas help you lose weight.
- Truvia and other sugar substitutes help you lose weight.
- Hormone D is a vitamin.
- That we can let untruths go unanswered without consequences, both intended and unintended.
- Calcium supplementation is good for you.
- Genetically modified organisms (GMOs) are good for you, and there will be no unintended consequences.
- Others I've already forgotten.

Okay, now let's review each and every one of these…

Mmm…maybe in the next book…or books. I've got a story to finish telling.

And next up are my very interesting meetings with some of the perpetrators of the aforementioned L-GAATs…

13
Nurse Marti and the Ada

December 21, 2011

As I drive to my appointment with Nurse Marti Sharon, I think to myself, *Finally I will get the answers I need*. Last night I made a list of questions so as not to miss anything.

I find a place to park right in front of the building where I will find my answers. I make my way up to the waiting room, where I sign in. My name is called, and I am ushered into Nurse Marti Sharon's office. It is small and cluttered, which actually makes it seem rather homey for a medical office.

Shortly, Nurse Marti Sharon comes in, apologizing for having a cold but explaining that she is only symptomatic and not contagious. She is very friendly and asks me a lot of questions.

I show her my journal and ask some questions of my own: "Why did my blood sugar level go down after I drank a beer? - Since a beer is full of carbohydrates, shouldn't my blood sugar level have risen?"

She answers, "No one knows why alcohol reduces blood sugar levels. But drinking alcohol is not recommended for obvious reasons."

I ponder the obvious reason out loud: "Because alcohol is a drug."

"That's right," Nurse Marti Sharon assures me and goes right on to the real reason I am here, which is to sell me on the idea of taking the approved drugs.

"Diabetes is not the end of the world," she says. "You and your doctor can manage it with proper medication." Seeing me frown at her mention of medication she offers, "You won't have to take insulin shots, ... well, not right away. ... Your doctor will probably start you off with Metformin."

Silence.

"I can give you your flu shot," she adds.

"No, thank you."

~·~

I go to my car. The battery is dead. I call a friend to come give me a jump start.

~·~

Ring. Ring. It is the receptionist from my doctor's office. She says I should go to a series of seven diabetes classes sponsored by the American Diabetes Association (ADA). I call the number she gives me in order to find out where and when.

As I drive to my first class with the ADA, I think to myself, *Finally I will get the answers I need.* Last night I made a list of questions so as not to miss anything.

I find a place to park right in front of the building where I will find my answers. I make my way up to the waiting room, where I sign in. My name is called, and I am ushered into a conference

Nurse Marti and the ADA

room with about six other diabetics, a small informal gathering with our group leader from the ADA, Ms. Ida.

Ms. Ida assures us that we can continue to eat whatever we want as long as we monitor our blood sugar levels and take our meds.

I ask skeptically, "Shouldn't we reduce our sugar consumption?"

She is quick to answer, "Why no. Sugar is just a carbohydrate. In fact, the ADA is trying to get sugar taken off of the food labels... because carbohydrates are already listed there. ...It's redundant."

No longer able to contain myself, I shout out before thinking, "I WANT TO KNOW HOW MUCH SUGAR IS IN THE FOOD I BUY!"

I probably overreacted. I have been fighting, unsuccessfully, to get genetically modified organisms, (GMO) "foods" labeled. GMOs are the same as Genetically Engineered Foods. They should be labeled as such. See more at https://www.facebook.com/justlabelit.

~·~

I go to my car. The battery is dead. I call a friend to come give me a jump start.

~·~

Needless to say, I do not go to the remaining six ADA classes. I am just going to have to continue reading books and researching on the Internet in order to learn anything about diabetes. It is obvious to me that the established medical system is not interested in finding out anything that might upset the status quo of selling drugs and selling sugar.

    In fact, I soon find out that refined white sugar is a drug. It is a drug more addictive than cocaine. Studies show brain scans of brains lit up by cocaine, and scans of brains lit up by sugar. They are identical.

~·~

I sell my old car for $1,500 and spend more time researching diabetes. I have a feeling that my studies are about to pay off...

14

Sir Lance-A-Lot, Finger-Pokin', and I Test Under "100"

December 27, 2011

Hear ye, hear ye, all ye whom do suffer the torture of lancing your fingers a lot, two to five times per day. In recognition of this unnatural woe, ye are hereby knighted, as I do dub thee Sir Lance-a-lot.

The size of the diabetes industry is $245 billion (it looks more impressive in numbers, $245,000,000,000.) per year. A big portion of that is the finger-pokin' segment of that industry. When you poke your finger to get blood to test, you are using two items each and every time:
1. A lance (you would think they could call it something less intimidating)
2. And a test strip.

These two items are not free. They are covered by most, if not all, health insurance plans, but someone has to pay for them.

Since you use one of each, each and every time you test your blood for your glucose level, then you are using…technically…a bunch of lances and strips.

The whole routine reminds me of the archaic medical practice of bloodletting. And before that it was blood sacrifice to the pagan gods. Seemingly, they have been replaced by Big Pharma.

Besides the cost in dollars, there is the cost in damage to your nerves, figuratively and literally. Your fingertips have very necessary nerve endings. When these nerve endings are continually poked and cut, they don't take it lying down. They retreat away from the surface of your skin. And the skin becomes thicker and harder to penetrate.

Even though I take neither insulin, nor any prescription drug, I have to poke a finger each and every time I test my blood glucose level.

In order to spread the misery around and not poke one finger more than any other, I make a map of my left hand and one of my right hand. Next I code my fingertips: L1, L2, etc. and R1, R2, etc. Then I keep a journal and record which finger I poke.

The diabetes industry has promised to develop and market a better method of testing, one that doesn't involve poking or bleeding. One idea is an ultrasound method of scanning your skin. Also in the works is a laser method. Another idea is to test the glucose in your saliva or tears.

With a better testing method, greater knowledge of diabetes would then follow. When we have to poke and bleed, we do that as little as necessary. With a non-invasive method, self-testing would be done more often. And we would learn more about diabetes: The effect of this food, or that exercise, or sleep, or whatever.

So far these advances are still in the research stage. Since they have been in research for years and years, it almost seems like a conspiracy to keep us in the dark about diabetes.

Is this an example of drug company profits in conflict with the interests of patients? And is it an example of the advancement of profit over the advancement of medical knowledge?

Sir Lance-A-Lot, Finger-Pokin', and I Test Under "100"

It's 5:21 p.m. time to poke my finger again.

There must be something wrong with my meter. It says that my blood glucose level is "87". Have I overdone something? I have never tested less than "100". I hear that low blood glucose is more dangerous than high blood glucose. Do I have hypoglycemia? Am I on the roller coaster of low glucose that will next shoot up to high glucose? Will I go into diabetic shock and coma?

Have I taken too much cinnamon? ...

15
Cinnamon

December 31, 2011, at midnight

The waitress brings us our coffee and I ask Melanie to pass the cinnamon. To pass the time, as we sip our hot coffees, I tell her a true story: "The US space program needed a zero gravity ball point pen, one that would write in space. As you may know, ballpoint pens work by gravity. They will not write upside down. So, NASA spent millions of dollars trying to develop the zero-gravity ballpoint pen."

"They should pay me. I can develop one." Melanie says, as she begins considering ways to make a zero-gravity ballpoint pen.

"Too late. The Russians have already solved the problem." I assure her.

"How?"

"They use a pencil."

~·~

Sometimes the simplest answer is the correct answer. Regarding diabetes, could cinnamon be the simple correct answer?

In a recent study published in *Diabetes Care* it is noted that...

"The results of this study demonstrate that intake of one, three, or six grams of cinnamon per day reduces serum glucose, triglyceride, LDL cholesterol, and total cholesterol in people with type 2 diabetes and suggest that the inclusion of cinnamon in the diet of people with type 2 diabetes will reduce risk factors associated with diabetes and cardiovascular diseases."

Cinnamon Improves Glucose and Lipids of People With Type 2 .., http://care.diabetesjournals.org/content/26/12/3215.long (accessed January 2, 2015).

In a recent 2014 study published in the peer reviewed *PLOS One* journal, it was concluded that...

"...cinnamon extract improved insulin action in the brain as well as brain activity and locomotion. This specific effect may represent an important central feature of cinnamon in improving insulin action in the brain, and mediates metabolic alterations in the periphery to decrease liver fat and improve glucose homeostasis."

Cinnamon extract improves insulin sensitivity in the brain .., http://www.ncbi.nlm.nih.gov/pubmed/24643026 (accessed January 2, 2015).

I have taken cinnamon capsules: one gram before each meal, every three or four hours, every day now for six weeks. And the results have astounded me. I feel healthier. I know that I am healthier, even before getting the official results from my doctor.

So tonight I celebrate. Tonight *we* celebrate. In one minute it will be midnight and the beginning of 2012, a new year and a renewed commitment to taking responsibility for our own health. No one knows your body and your health better than you. And no one knows what your body needs better than your own body. If given half a chance, your body will tell you what it needs to be healthy. At times your body will crave what is good for it. Listen to it. Use your intuition and your good judgment. This is true hope based upon well-placed faith.

Faith in my journals, tables, and charts…oh my…

PART III
2012 AND 2013

16

Journals, Tables, and Charts, Oh My

January 19, 2012, at midnight

The house is quite. It's late, well past my bedtime. The kitchen table is cluttered with graph paper, pencils of different colors, and rulers. I am preparing tables from my journal and then charts from my tables.

I have again managed to wait until the last minute to prepare for an important meeting, my meeting with Doctor Smith, my primary care physician.

That meeting is 11:00 a.m. tomorrow, and I want to present the results of my last nine weeks in an informative, organized, and efficient way. Since I am still a geeky tax accountant, what I have done is to:

1. Record in my journals.
2. Summarize in my tables. and
3. Analyze in my charts.

G. E. Frazier, CHC

I select eight charts that show, chronologically and sequentially, the fact that my blood glucose reading is higher in the morning than it is later in the day.

Therefore, the following eight charts prove that I am Dawn Phenomenon:

Journals, Tables, and Charts, Oh My

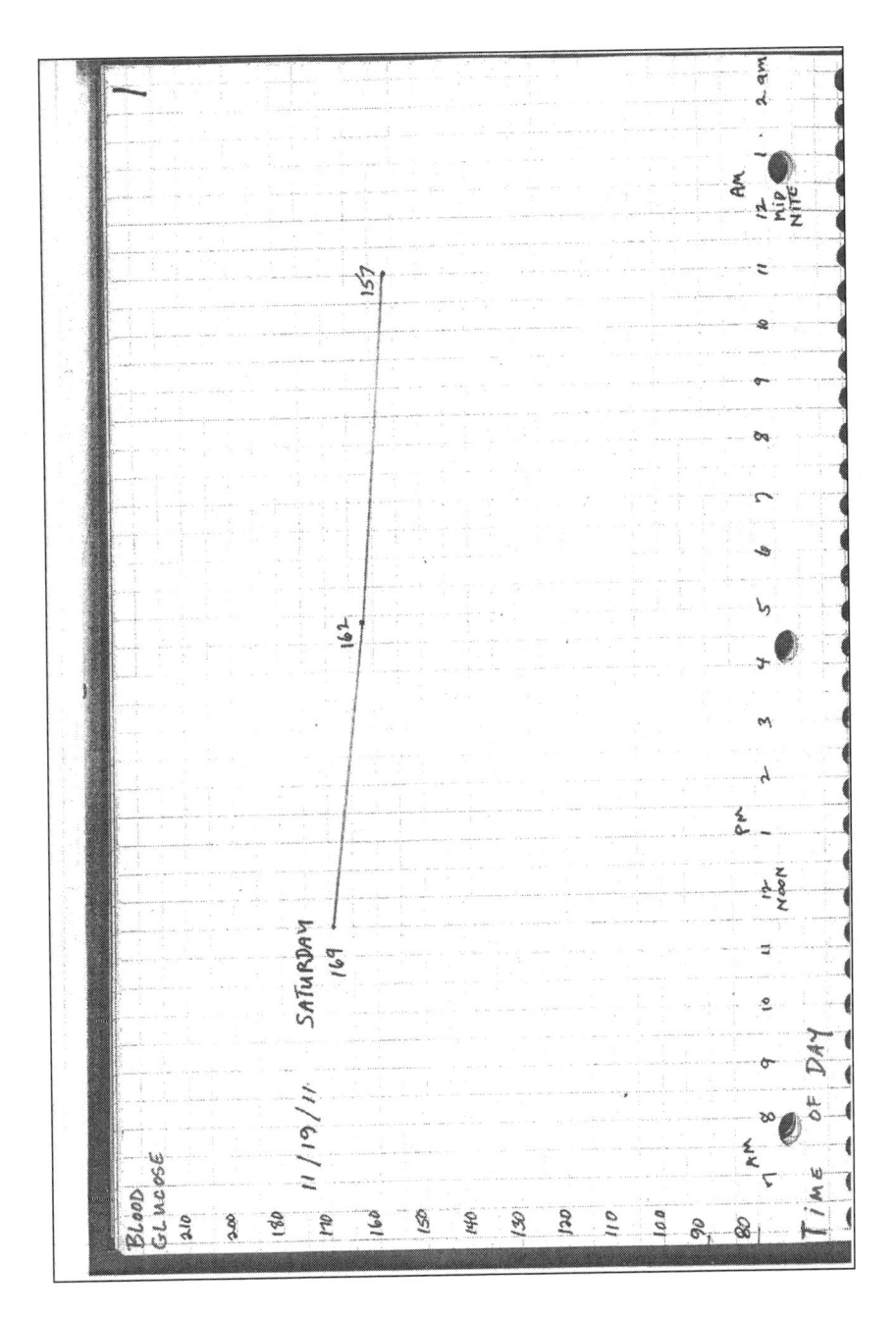

Chart 1

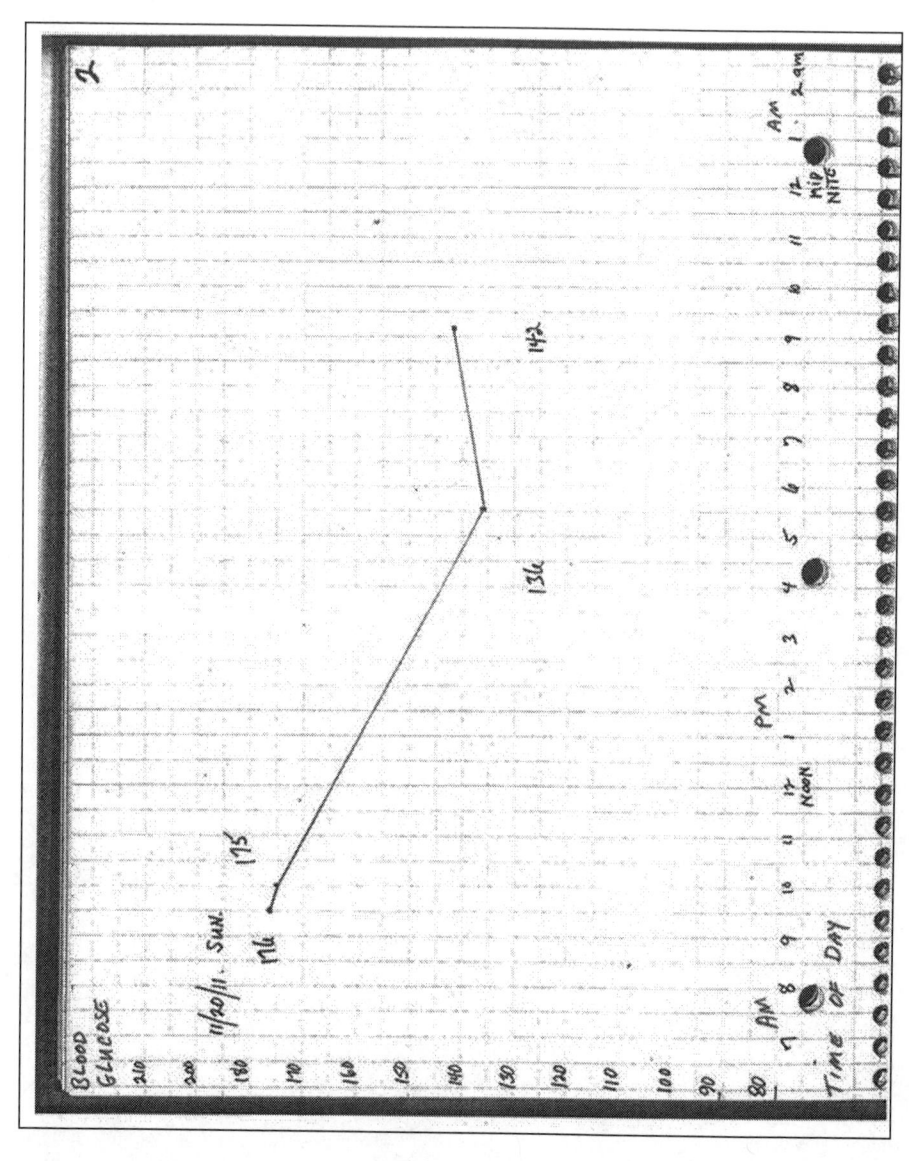

Chart 2

Journals, Tables, and Charts, Oh My

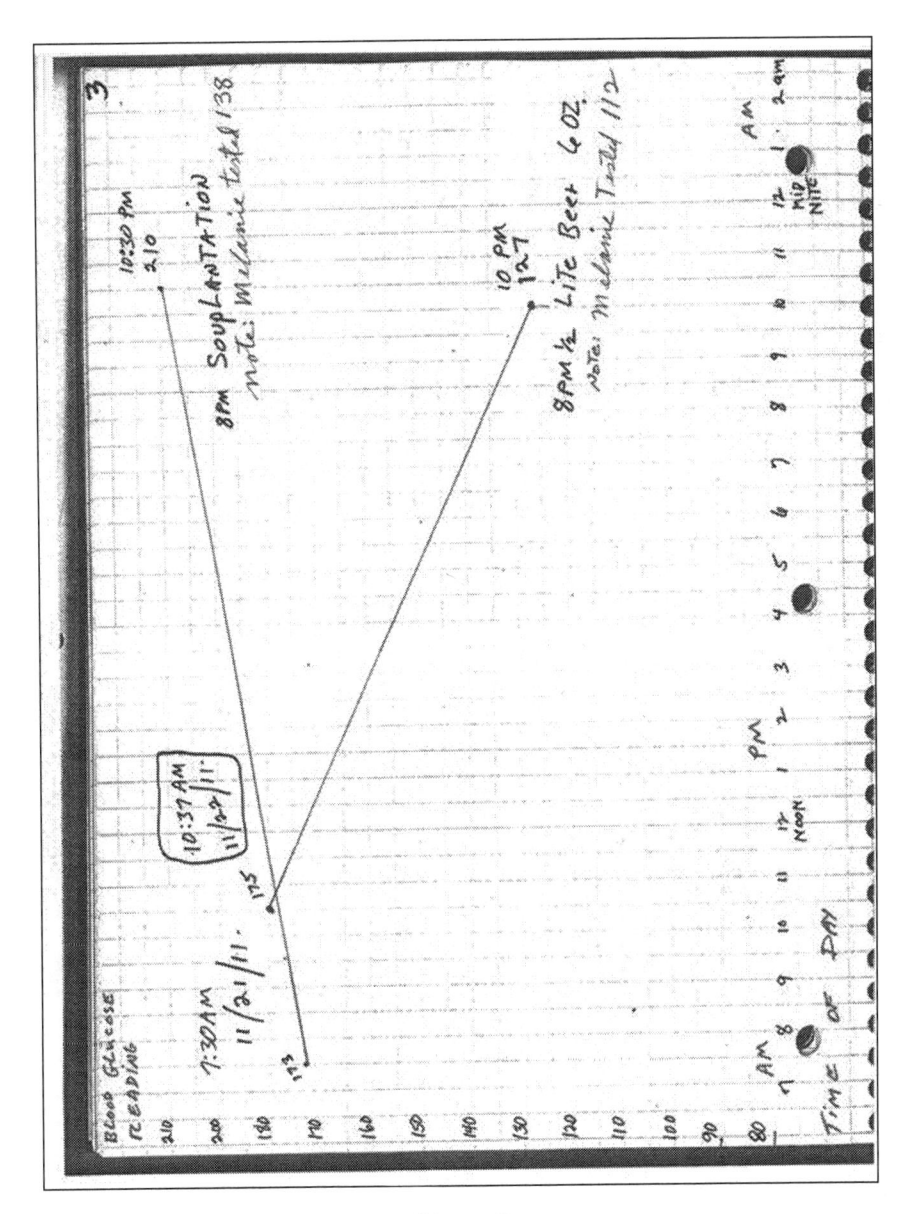

Chart 3

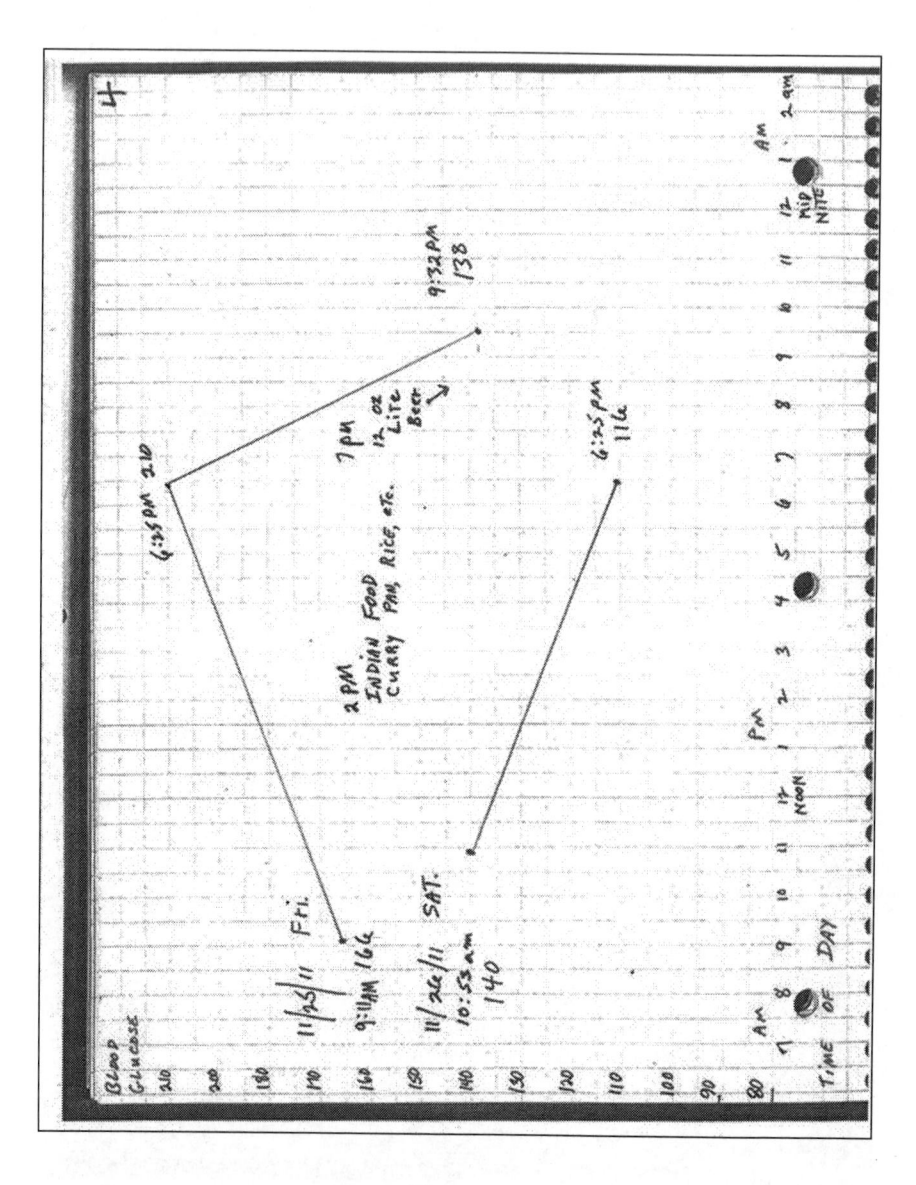

Chart 4

Journals, Tables, and Charts, Oh My

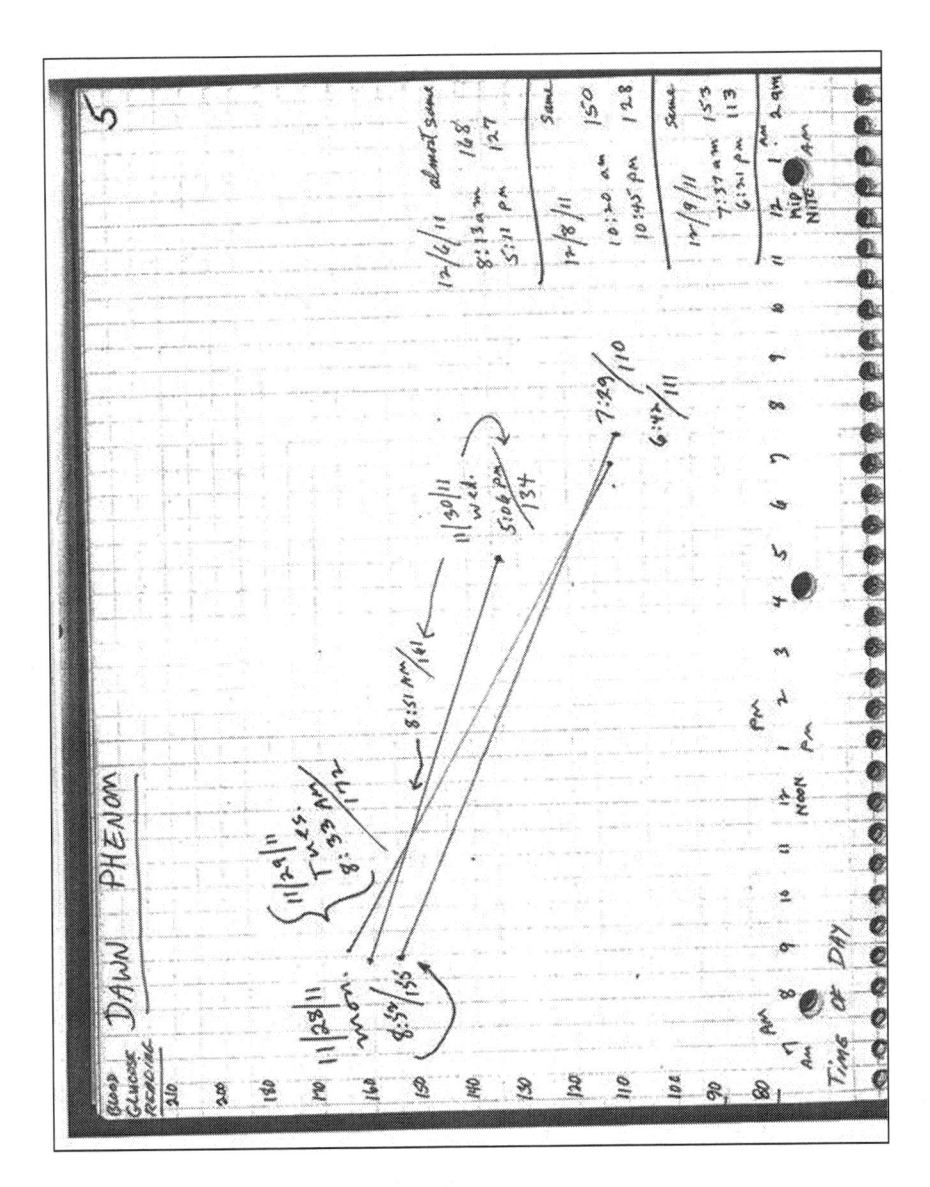

Chart 5

101

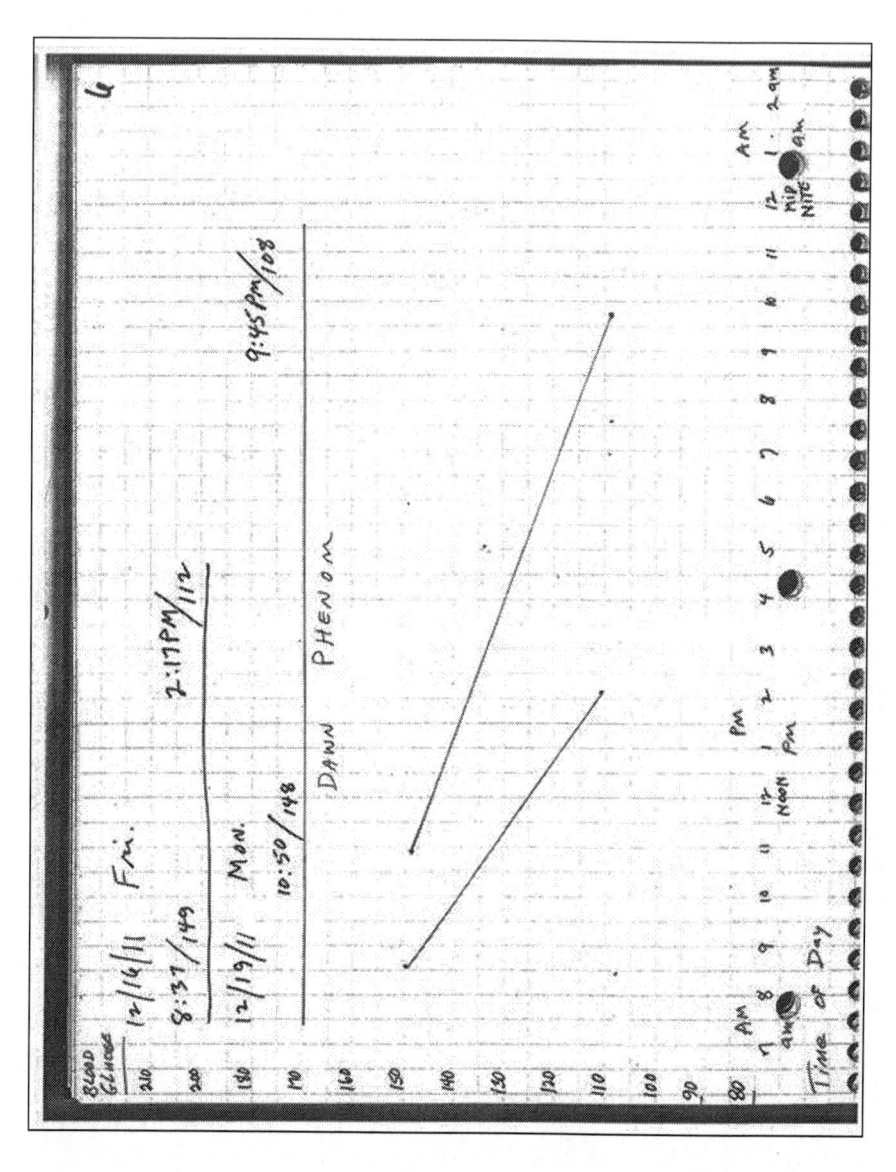

Chart 6

Journals, Tables, and Charts, Oh My

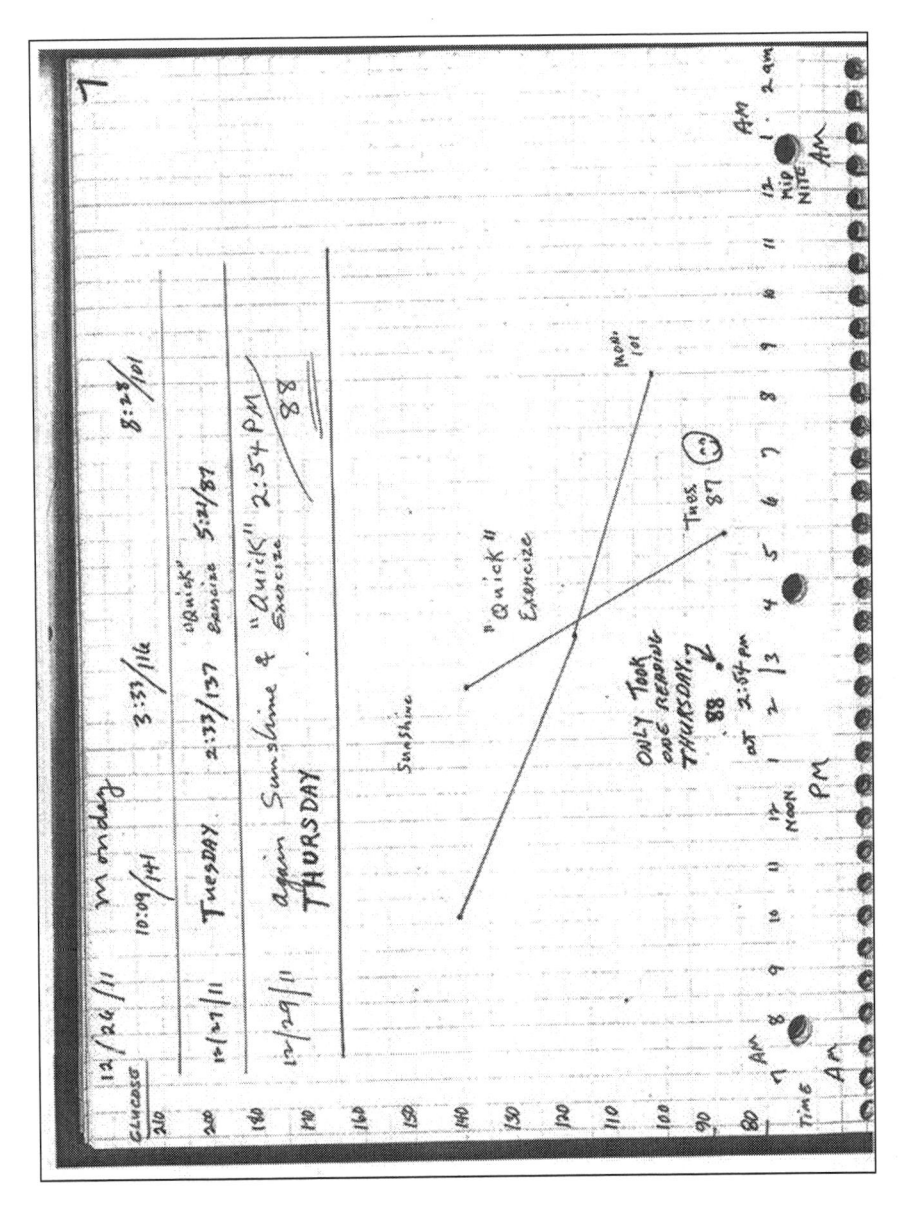

Chart 7

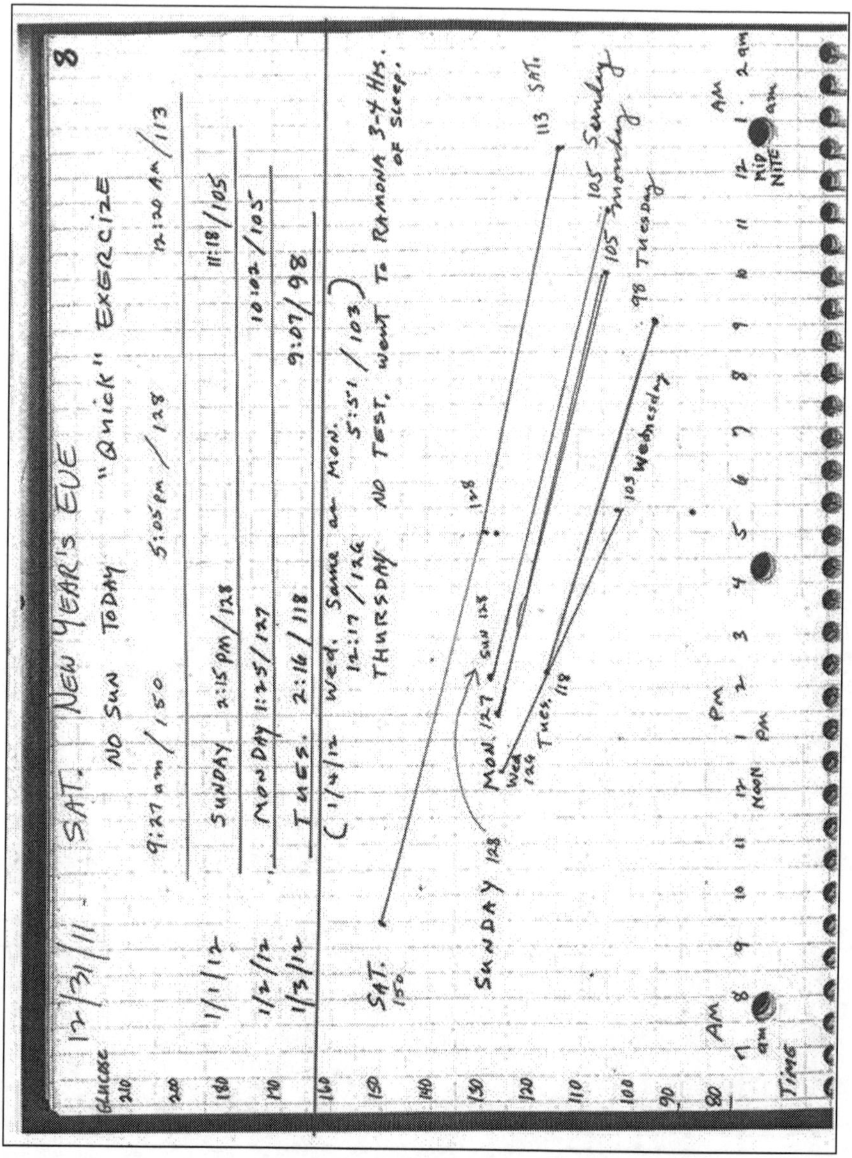
12/31/11 - SAT. New Year's Eve
NO SUN TODAY
"Quick" EXERCIZE
9:27 am / 150
5:05 pm / 128
12:20 AM / 113
1/1/12 SUNDAY 2:15 PM/128
11:18/105
1/2/12 MONDAY 1:25/127
10:02/105
1/3/12 TUES. 2:16/118
9:07/98
1/4/12 Wed. Same as Mon.
12:17/126
5:51/103
THURSDAY NO TEST. WENT TO RAMONA 3-4 Hrs. OF SLEEP.

Chart 8

Journals, Tables, and Charts, Oh My

Next I compute daily averages of blood glucose readings and plot them on the following charts 9A and 9B. These two charts show a definite downward trend from "192" down to "91." The reading of "91" is well below "100" which is considered normal.

Chart 9A goes from 11/19/11 through 12/27/11. Chart 9B continues on from 12/27/11 through 1/19/12. To me, this proves that I am cured of diabetes.

The line across the middle of these two charts is drawn at "130." Nine weeks ago that was my goal. I have reached my goal of "130" and exceeded it.

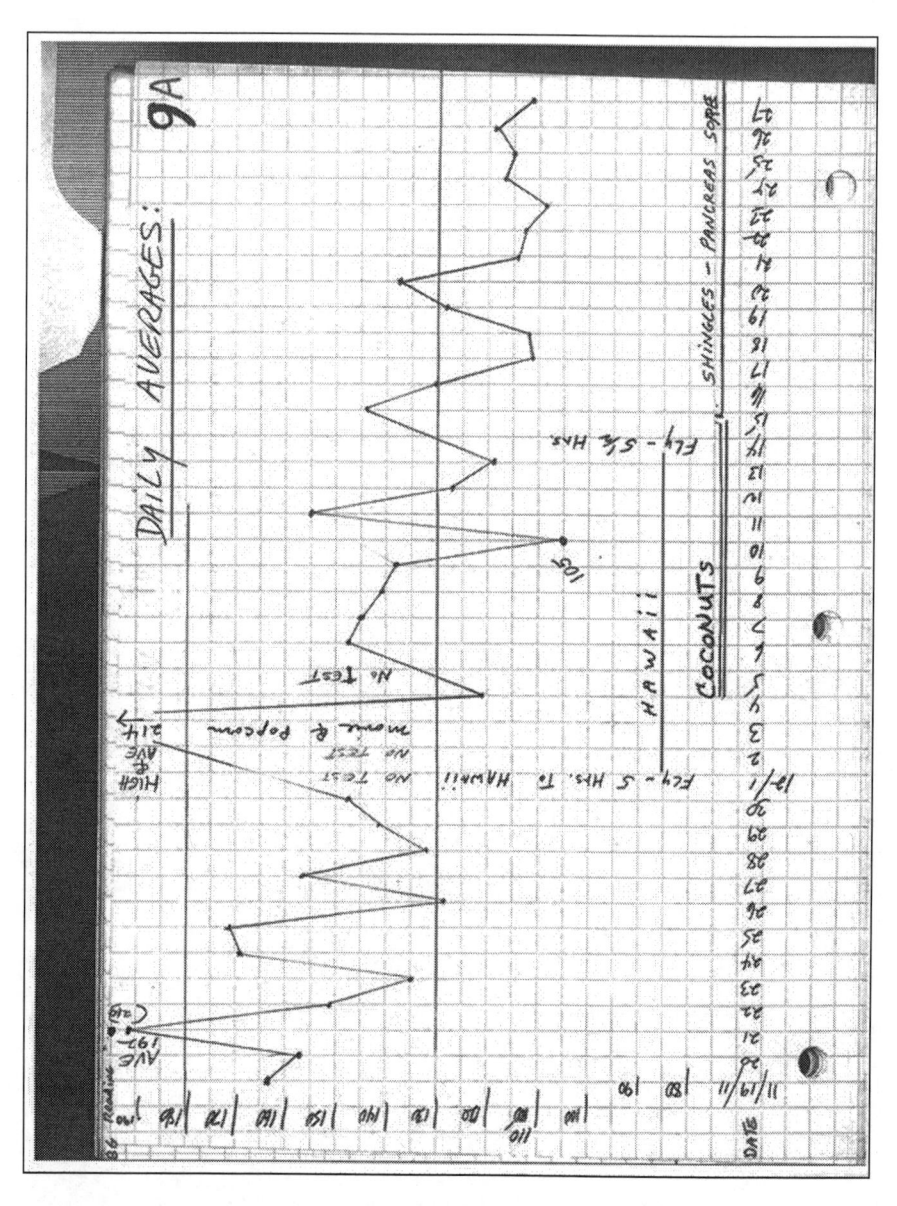

Chart 9A

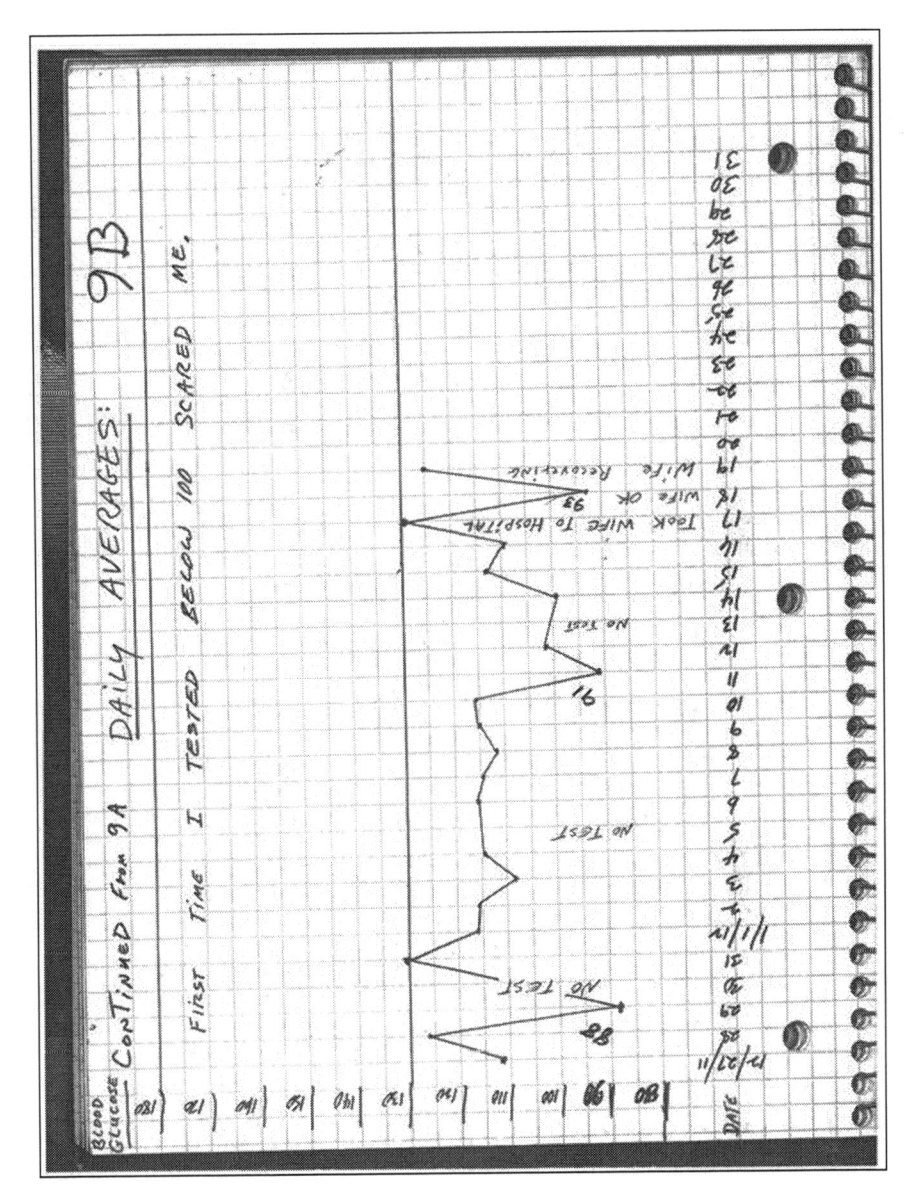

Chart 9B

I feel that I am ready. Armed with these ten charts, I will go to my doctor's appointment and discuss with my doctor how taking cinnamon has allowed my body to cure itself of diabetes without having to take dangerous prescription drugs.

I am positive that Dr. Smith will want to know how I did it, so he can help his other patients. Maybe he will want to write a research paper based upon my findings.

Yes, I am ready to help my doctor help others. I am prepared for tomorrow's doctor's visit…

17
My Final Doctor's Visit

January 20, 2012, at 5:20 a.m.

Maria, the receptionist from Dr. Smith's office, has faithfully given me the standard patient instructions for a diabetic. I am not to eat or drink anything this morning because the doctor will want to take my fasting blood glucose reading.

I get up at 5:20 a.m. and drink eight ounces of water because I know that the doctor will also want a urine sample.

Last night was a good night's sleep. Even though it was only five hours, it was five continuous hours of sound sleep. I am well rested, and that is good because I have a busy day. I am super excited about meeting with my doctor, so he can see that I am cured of an incurable disease.

At 6:55 a.m. I'm at my gym to exercise.

At 8:00 a.m. I stop by my office to photocopy my ten charts.

At precisely 11:00 a.m. I open my doctor's front door and enter his office. Receptionist Maria asks me to take a seat in the waiting room. After a while, I am escorted to an exam room, where the nurse pokes my finger and gets a blood glucose reading of 135. Next, she takes my blood pressure. It is 139 over eighty-four with a pulse rate of seventy-one. She looks in vain for a vein and finally finds one. So she can draw my blood to send to a lab for an A1c test. This test will give us my blood glucose number that number will represent my average blood glucose level over the past three months.

"I can give you your flu shot while you wait for the doctor."
"No thanks."

~·~

REGARDING FLU SHOTS:

As reported by Sylvia Booth Hubbard, Writer:
"A Johns Hopkins scientist has issued a blistering report on influenza vaccines in the *British Medical Journal* (BMJ). Peter Doshi, PhD., charges that although the vaccines are being pushed on the public in unprecedented numbers, they are less effective and cause more side effects than alleged by the Centers for Disease Control and Prevention (CDC). Further, says Doshi, the studies that underlie the CDC's policy of encouraging most people to get a yearly flu shot are often low quality studies that do not substantiate the official claims." - A Johns Hopkins scientist has issued a blistering report on .., http://www.yournaturalhealth.com/natural_health_news/2013/10/a-johns-hopkins-scientist-has.html (accessed January 3, 2015).

As an interesting aside, the Internet is reporting that the CDC just issued an apology for the lack of effectiveness of this year's flu vaccine.

Not to mention that all vaccinations contain mercury. And there is no safe amount of mercury that should be put into your body.

~·~

My Final Doctor's Visit

It is almost noon, and I haven't eaten anything. And the last hour has been spent sitting in the doctor's office, inactive. Both things are conducive to raising my blood glucose level.

Doctor Smith enters the room briskly. "Hello. How are you today?"

"I am great. And I have some charts to show you."

"You have? Well your blood pressure is high."

"I have 'white-coat syndrome.' My blood pressure is usually in the 120s at home."

"Let me take it again." He does, and now it is over 150.

"Your cholesterol is high too. I am going to put you on statins…as well as blood thinner." Dr. Smith has his prescription pad out again and adds, "Metformin and…"

"Doctor, shouldn't you wait for the results of today's A1c blood test first?"

Finally I see evidence of thought, rather than the prejudgments and preprogrammed solutions that Dr. Smith was offering before.

This is my opening and I jump in with both feet. "I am feeling much better. My blood glucose readings have been coming down to where they are now at normal levels for a Dawn Phenomenon."

Dr. Smith acknowledges, "You do look healthier."

"Do you know the term Dawn Phenomenon?" I ask.

"No." Dr. Smith admits with a curious puzzled look on his face.

"Then you will be interested in these charts. They demonstrate what it is. Look right here: See the blood glucose level is highest in the morning until I eat something. Then it stops going up and goes down the rest of the day."

My hopes rise as Dr. Smith examines my charts and says, "There is a definite downward trend."

However, after a brief pause, Dr. Smith states in a tone that denotes finality, "But it is the averages that count." As he hands my charts back to me.

I am not giving up without a sustained "college try." So I persist: "Charts 9A and 9B are daily averages."

Dr. Smith has experienced more college than I have; he merely changes the subject. "Are you feeling depressed?"

That question hits me like a nail puncturing a rubber tire; I am now completely deflated. There is no use. His mind is made up. I just have to wait for the results of today's A1c test, and that could take several days.

~·~

Then, just three days later, while at work in my office, I was surprised by receptionist Maria's phone call:

"Hello. This is Dr. Smith's office calling. The doctor says, 'Congratulations. Keep up the good work.'"

"Oh, hello...what...uh, thank you...what was my A1c reading?"

"6.1."

An A1c reading is an average of blood glucose levels over the last three-months. Therefore, my current actual blood glucose level today has to be less than 6.1!

Follow my logic here. If nine weeks ago my A1c reading was 7.8, which it was, then those high levels nine weeks ago are included in my three month average number today. So an A1c reading now of 6.1 means to me, that my actual blood glucose level today is at a level below 6.1.

Since an A1c reading of 6.0 is "normal" ... No diabetes.... I no longer have diabetes.

"Whoo hoo!"

My Final Doctor's Visit

G. E. Frazier: no more type II diabetes (insulin resistance), just Dawn Phenomenon. I do not blame Dr. Smith for thinking I had diabetes. It is the fasting test for diabetes that I blame. As a Dawn Phenomenon, you must insist upon the A1c test before taking any medicine for diabetes.

My A1c was 7.8; then nine weeks later my A1c is 6.1.

I lost forty-five pounds, and seven inches from around my waist.

My cholesterol came down to ninety-eight. (One hundred is good.)

Also, my blood pressure eventually came down to an average of 110.

What can I do now with my extraordinary success in beating an incurable disease?

I continue my studies…

18
Further Study and I Find a New Career

July 1, 2012

When researching on the Internet, it is easy to go off on a tangent. You can become sidetracked on irrelevant subjects. I know I wasted a lot of time doing just that. Then so much information is outdated. You can get confused when seemingly good information contradicts other good information.

So, I am sitting at my computer getting brain fog when it hits me: ... What I need is a structured course of study. By taking a formal course, I will be able to find and cover the relevant information in less time.

Research of the available courses leads me to choose the international Institute for Integrative Nutrition (IIN).

The day after April 15, I will be finished with the annual tax season work of preparing tax returns. During the month of May, I catch up on all the things I put off doing until after April 15. Then in June, I rest. So there is plenty of time for me to go back to school in June or July ... next year.

What? Well ... I don't want to rush into anything. I mean, I do feel great, and I want to share my knowledge and experience with others.

Can't I just write a book?

It is 2012. I have reached the big "seven-o." I have been practicing tax accounting for forty years. Maybe it is time for a change. Plus Obama wants the IRS to administer ObamaCare. That means the IRS will expect tax accountants to administer ObamaCare. That is something I did not sign up for. I mean, I do not agree. I believe ObamaCare to be neither, good for me, good for my clients, nor good for the country. So for that reason, alone, I cannot get my heart into the coming tax season.

~·~

Mrs. Joy calls. "Mr. Frazier? Bill died. What do I do…with the IRS, I mean?"

"Oh no, I am so sorry. Bill was so healthy and active. I mean he swam two miles a day…in the ocean."

Mrs. Joy agrees. "It was unexpected. He just died in his sleep."

Too many of my tax clients are getting sick, and many are dying. They have more health issues than tax issues. They need "health saving" more than they need "tax saving." I make a decision: I will try to help them achieve good health and long lives by offering my services as a certified health coach (CHC).

Becoming a certified health coach will take twelve months of hard study. I need to sell my tax practice in order to devote the time necessary to learn enough to help others.

I find two enrolled agents who are willing to help my clients with their tax problems. I will continue to work as many tax seasons as is necessary until I am sure that these two can serve my tax clients well. Many clients have been with me for forty years or more. (Also as an aside, notice that it takes two enrolled agents to replace one, me.)

Further Study and I Find a New Career

That settled, on July 1, 2013, I am off to school to begin my second career as a health coach. I believe that health coaching is the future of effective disease prevention.

School is exciting. I surprise myself at how quickly I get back into the groove of going to class, taking tests, etc.

~·~

In case you are interested in learning over one hundred diet theories and how to integrate them into the best custom diet for each individual, then contact http://integrativenutrition.com

If at school you would like for me to be your accountability partner and sponsor, I would be happy to do that for you. Just mention that you are being referred by gfrazier2 - (class of July, 2013).

It is a twelve-month class – my class graduates July, 2014....

PART IV
2014 AND WAY BEYOND

19
Graduation

July 1, 2014

School was actually fun, and I earned the certified health coach (CHC) designation. I will put out my shingle, as they say. My practice will specialize in disease prevention and wellness support for:
- Dawn Phenomenon,
- Pre-diabetics,
- diabetics,
- weight loss,
- eating for health and longevity, and
- super health and wellness.

And of course, I still want to write my book. Semi-retired, I now have time on my hands, and so I sign up for a writing class. Eager to help as many people as possible, I decide that finishing this book would be the best use of my time in order to reach as many people as possible.

I will always make time for coaching a Dawn Phenomenon. We can interact over the Internet with Skype or FaceTime.

My group classes are on the evils of addictive processed sugar, other processed foods, and now the dangers of engineered "foods," GMOs.

There is an Internet-TV show in the works. In the meantime, check out my website, blog, Twitter, Facebook page, and Amazon page.

On the back burner is an idea for a diabetic's boot camp, a place where diabetics can get away and concentrate on healthy living. This would be an attempt to recreate my Hawaiian getaway that helped me so much.

~·~

Large companies are finding that they benefit from educating their employees about the healthiness of mindful eating. Many employers hire health coaches to give classes and workshops to their employees on practical ways to get the most nutrition for their food dollars.

Both employees and employers benefit.

Employers find that sick days are reduced thus saving money directly, and indirectly by an increase in productive work from healthy, energized employees. The money saved can be substantial. As a recovering accountant, I can compute that.

~·~

Mainly I want to see diabetes as a thing of the past. With your help we can do it. The healthy habits in this book can help you live a healthful life well into your hundreds.

May you die young... late in life!

~·~

In this book, I state my opinions based upon what I have seen, heard, and read, all filtered through my seventy-two years of observation and experience. The opinions expressed in this book are my own. If you have a different opinion, let's discuss it; I am always open to learning more. If you have questions or constructive comments, do not hesitate to contact me. I will be happy to talk with you.

The ideas in this book worked for me. I encourage you to experiment with them as I did. Make them your own. Nothing here is being prescribed to you. I am not a medical doctor. I am a certified health coach, an integrative nutrition health coach, and a member of the International Association for Health Coaches (IAHC). To personally coach you to your best ever health and wellness would be my pleasure and an honor.

~·~

This is not the end of my voyage. I must begin a journey now to learn how to promote this book, so that my story can help as many people as possible. If you have information that will help another person, you have a moral obligation to make that information available to that person. I have a moral obligation to make this information available to as many other people as possible.

To doctors: Now that you know about the Dawn Phenomenon, you will not misdiagnose the Dawn Phenomenon as diabetic.

Now consider the possibility that Dawn Phenomenon is the normal healthy condition for everyone. As we have seen in this book, the Dawn Phenomenon is not automatically diabetic. Rather the Dawn Phenomenon displays the traits of super wellness. Maybe eating too much processed sugar has made us sick. Maybe our diet has damaged our livers/pancreases to the point that our glucose/insulin "dance" is out of balance.

I recommend that everyone aspire to be a Dawn Phenomenon of super wellness.

And to all you super healthy Dawn Phenomenon everywhere: Know that you are normal, in fact beyond normal, special, because every morning at 3:00 a.m. your body, specifically your healthy liver, prepares you to be better able to compete for your benefit and the benefit of your loved ones.

Trust your body to know what to do and when to do it. Feed yourself nutritious foods. This gives your body what it needs in order to do its job of keeping you healthy.

You are the only one with the power to change your life. Remember, I'm not telling you what to do; your body knows what to do. First, I coach you to listen to your body. Then together we set your own goals. I coach you on how to break down your goals into manageable chunks with realistic deadlines. Finally, I hold you accountable to your own plan.

Deadlines! I just love deadlines. I especially like the whooshing sound they make as they go passing by.

So before that final deadline comes whooshing by, please remember these principles:
- Honor your ancestors.
- Poor health causes disease.
- Be grateful.
- Biodiversity.
- Trust your intuition.
- Trust your body.
- Eat the rainbow (a variety of foods) with balance.
- Question authority.
- Substitute the good for the bad.
- Eat whole foods and chew them well.
- Buy organic, support your local farmers.

- Take rest and relaxation. If you slip up, don't beat yourself up.
- First: do no harm, do *not* eat processed sugar, purified salt, or processed foods of any kind. Moderation in all things.
- Read labels. Buy organic to avoid genetically modified organisms (GMOs).
- To lose bad fat, eat good fat.
- Get your ions, practice earthing.
- Try oil pulling.
- Question the L-GAAT, Lies Generally Accepted As True.
- Consider cinnamon.
- Keep a journal.
- Avoid all vaccinations.
- If your fasting blood glucose level is high, insist on an A1c test.
- Continue your education.
- And above all: Be thankful that you are one of the 20 percent of people who have inherited the energy, and the super health and wellness, of a Dawn Phenomenon.

It is my contention that the Dawn Phenomenon is the normal healthy state of being. And that anyone can be Dawn Phenomenon if they try.

Are you down with Dawn Phenomenon? Then take these actions while they are still fresh in your mind.
1. Get eight hours sleep every night.
2. Upon waking do twenty minutes of intermittent exercise every other day.
3. Within thirty minutes of exercise, or waking, eat a high-protein breakfast.
4. Trust your body.

5. Eat a variety of fresh natural local seasonal organic whole foods. Prepare them using the least amount of heat necessary.
6. Be spiritual, optimistic, and energetic. (You are energy.)
7. Question authority. (It's also above as one of the principles.)
8. Guard your liberty.
9. Demand reasonable proof, and check it out on the Internet.
10. Be a truth seeker. Join the health-and-wellness revolution.

Commit to a six-month Dawn Phenomenon protocol, because in a few days your memory of this book will fade and leave. If you are not on board, you will regret it. Oh, maybe not today! Maybe not tomorrow! But soon! ...And forever!

EPILOGUE

"If people let government decide what foods they eat and what medicines they take, their bodies will soon be in as sorry a state as are the souls (lives) of those who live under tyranny."
–Thomas Jefferson

You are encouraged to accept responsibility for your own health and happiness and to reject the government's attempts to control your life with ObamaCare. ObamaCare is centralized, top-down, socialized medicine. We don't like trickle-down economics, so why would we like trickle-down health care? I believe with all my heart that ObamaCare was written to protect the status quo of power and profit currently enjoyed by the large insurance companies and Big Pharma. ObamaCare will not give us more health care, but less.

ObamaCare: repeal it, defund it, and eliminate governmental interference in your health and happiness—because ObamaCare is institutionalized bureaucracy, and institutionalized bureaucracy stifles innovations.

You have a divine right to health and wellness. "Divine" means that your right comes from God, not from the government. The government can only get in the way with taxes and regulations. The gift of health and wellness is everyone's divine right. Ask and you shall receive. Knock and the door will be opened for you. Focus and ask the right question and nothing is impossible. Mountains will be moved…meaning burdensome problems will be lifted…if you but ask the right questions.

Besides, now there is a better alternative to ObamaCare: the better alternative is to join the wellness revolution and hire a certified health coach. As an Integrative Nutrition Certified Health Coach, I am trained to help you to "ask the right questions!"

REFERENCES AND CONCLUDING THOUGHTS

The following are the three citations on the 1993 scientific study that should have changed medicine for the better and made ObamaCare unnecessary. Read these for proof that disease does not cause poor health, rather it is poor health that causes disease.

> Ford ES, Bergmann MM, Kroger J, Schienkiewitz A, Weikert C, Boeing H. "Healthy living is the best revenge: findings from the European Prospective Investigation Into Cancer and Nutrition-Potsdam study." *Arch Intern Med.* 2009 Aug 10;169(15):1355–62.

> Kvaavik E, Batty GD, Ursin G, Huxley R, Gale CR. "Influence of individual and combined health behaviors on total and cause-specific mortality in men and women: the United Kingdom health and lifestyle survey." *Arch Intern Med.* 2010;170:711–8.

> McCullough ML, Patel AV, Kushi LH, Patel R, Willett WC, Doyle C, Thun MJ, Gapstur SM. "Following cancer prevention guidelines reduces risk of cancer, cardiovascular disease, and all-cause mortality." *Cancer Epidemiol Biomarkers Prev.* 2011;20:1089–97.

Diabetes data has been taken from many sources including: Statistics About Diabetes - Data from the National Diabetes Statistics Report, 2014 (released June 10, 2014) Overall Numbers, Diabetes and Prediabetes Prevalence: the number of people in (the

USA) who are reported to have (diabetes or prediabetes): In 2012, 29.1 million Americans, or 9.3% of the population, had diabetes. (In 2010 the figures were 25.8 million and 8.3%.) Prediabetes: In 2012, 86 million Americans age 20 and older had prediabetes, a condition in which blood glucose levels are higher than normal, but are not high enough for a diagnosis of diabetes. People with prediabetes are at increased risk for developing type 2 diabetes and for heart disease and stroke. Other names for prediabetes are impaired glucose tolerance and *impaired fasting glucose.X*; this is up from 79 million in 2010. http://www.diabetes.org/diabetes-basics/statistics/#sthash.NGxoJAec.dpuf - According to the American Diabetes Association, http://www.diabetes.org/diabetes-basics/statistics/ accessed 12/27/14.

I wonder how many Dawn Phenomenon are wrongly included above in the category: "*impaired fasting glucose.X?*"

If medical doctors would stop listening to the drug companies long enough to read about these studies, maybe they would realize that ObamaCare is more of the same: the wrong direction in medicine.

The Affordable Health Care Act is neither affordable nor health care. Again I say, mostly to the U. S. Congress, grow a pair and repeal it. Defund it. Shut down the government, if necessary, anything to stop the Affordable Health Care Act.

In fact, let's have a day without government: one day with no federal taxes, no federal regulations (except for national security of course: military, border patrol, etc.). But everything else the federal government does is unnecessary.

As government, itself, said, during the recent government shut down: *We are closing down, please notice.*

Hardly anyone did.

~·~

REFERENCES AND CONCLUDING THOUGHTS

For a good explanation as to why today's medical system is a failed system, see the Natural News website at http://www.naturalnews.com/. It is dedicated to explaining why mechanistic medicine is a failed system of medicine. As reported by NNW, most modern-day scientists do not believe that any vitamin, mineral, or food has any biological effect whatsoever on the human body, other than providing calories, sugars, proteins, fiber and fat. This wildly delusional belief is enshrined in the FDA's regulatory framework and is practiced throughout hospitals and health clinics across the planet.

Yet, this belief is inconsistent with the facts. For example, how can minerals play no role in human health when elements like sodium, potassium, magnesium, and calcium are necessary for the most fundamental chemical and electrical processes of muscle neurology? (And, as we are finding: we may be getting too much calcium.) Minerals are necessary for over a trillion bodily functions. ACTION: Eat green vegetables with butter, unpurified sea salt, or rock salt, and garlic. They taste so good too.

Check references, ask the Universal Mind, and trust your intuition. Ask questions. Have faith that the answers will come. Take part in the health-and-wellness revolution that is presently uplifting our human civilization.

Before you make any changes based upon this book, whether to your diet, lifestyle, or any area of your life, first check the appropriateness of such changes for you with your own health practitioner.

Life-changing health coaching is available. The first step is to contact a Certified Health Coach (CHC). If you like my informal style, go to my web site, GEFrazier.com and sign up for a free 50 minute health history evaluation session. Next fill out the health history form you'll find there on my web site under "CONNECT" at "HEALTH FORMS." You can fill out, and submit the form, right on my website. And I will get back to you. Then you and I will talk. You ask me questions about the process. I ask you questions about your health. When I feel that I can definitely help you, and, you feel comfortable too. Then together we will customize a health coaching program of continued sessions so we can meet twice a month. That's all there is to it. I am in San Diego, California. However, it doesn't matter where you are as long as you have a phone or the Internet. We health coaches are able to work over the phone, Skype, or FaceTime. I will look after you. Guaranteed.

I want to leave you with a word about anti-aging: dumb. It is just dumb. You are going to age. The question is, will you do so gracefully and remain healthy?

Longevity is possible. Even though I write about the genes that evolved down to us, we are not slaves to our genes. Someday, we humans will figure out how to master the environment of our genes, so that our genes will change themselves in ways that beneficially serve us, which is the new science of epigenetics. If this interests you, find out more by googling Dr. Bruce Lipton.

I will leave you with this concluding thought:

When it is my time to go, I want to die peacefully in my sleep like my grandfather... not yelling and screaming, like the passengers in his car.

~·~~·~

~·~

ABOUT THE AUTHOR

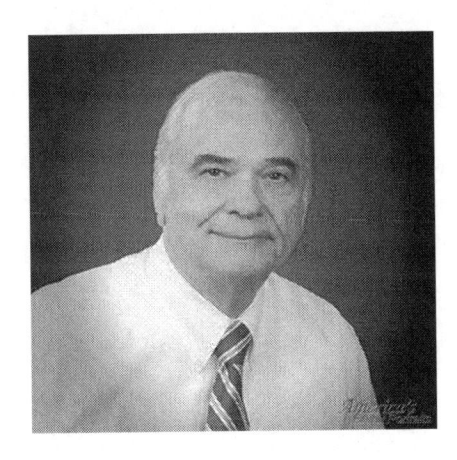

G. E. Frazier, CHC, is a certified health coach and graduate of the Institute for Integrative Nutrition. He holds a BS in accounting from San Diego State University and was a tax accountant for forty-three years. Now, instead of researching tax law, he researches health and wellness. He practices in San Diego, where he lives with his loving wife, Melanie.

On November 17, 2011, Frazier was diagnosed with diabetes. However, refusing to accept that diagnosis, he discovered his true condition as "dawn phenomenon," and cured his diabetes in nine weeks. This book chronicles his unusual nine week journey and shares what he has learned so that others can join the wellness revolution as well.